Listening To Life

Words of Encouragement, Support

And Comfort

By

Sylvia Payne Swanson

Additional Printing 2024
Printed in U.S.A. and Other

ISBN 979-8-9856713-1-5

Cover Design By the Studio of Curtis N. Swanson
Author Photo by Curtis N. Swanson
Vero Beach, FL 32962

Contents

Chapter 1 - Nature

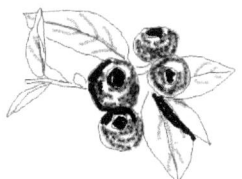

A MESSAGE FROM WILD BLUEBERRIES

Have you ever had the fun of picking wild blueberries? I grew up in the Midwest where they flourish and, if my brother and I picked enough, mom would turn them into a pie. It was hard to pick enough because instant gratification took over, so we ate as we picked, immediately enjoying their sweetness. As an adult I am aware of more than their sweet flavor. Nutritionists say these little berries are packed with important nutrients, including the highest level of antioxidants in any food. Domestic berries are also nourishing, but do not contain the same high level of nutrients as wild blueberries.

Wild blueberries have a history thousands of years old, and have survived because of their ability to adapt to climate change, and their capacity for recovering after trauma. Many plants are eliminated by fire, but the wild blueberry plant can be completely burned away and still sprout and regrow right up through the ashes. In fact, it will come back even stronger and healthier because, as it grows, it uses the nutrients in the ashes to feed its new growth. The plant doesn't just survive, it thrives after being destroyed!

How many of us have had the unexpected (fire) catch us by surprise. It's the phone call alerting us that a loved one has been in a serious accident, or the announcement from our trusted spouse that they are in love with someone else. It's the diagnosis that calls us to look at our mortality, or the loss of a needed job. Any loss can make us feel like our whole world has changed, and we have hit rock bottom.

The best thing we can do for ourselves is not to pretend everything is okay when it isn't. There's no prize for suffering secretly. Uttering the magic word "help" opens the pathway for support, understanding, and love to guide us into all we need to survive and thrive. When we feel we're in the valley, we sometimes wish we were on the mountaintop, but on the mountain top the air is thin and it's hard to breath. We can only stand still and try not to fall. A nourishing river runs in the valley and that is where the power to overcome is found.

Author Glennon Doyle Melton writes, "We want to be on the mountaintops, but we are not called to be victorious. We're called to be wise, strong and kind. We are admired on the mountaintops, but we are beloved in the valleys."[1] It's when we are called to unbecome everything we thought we were and start over again, that we do our hardest but most essential work. The pain of loss brings uncertainty, and our instinct is to scramble away from it and get back to what is familiar. But rushing out of the valley means we miss gathering the wisdom, strength, courage and kindness needed to take us through surviving to thriving.

Like the wild blueberry growing through the ashes of what was, we can sit by the river and claim its gifts. Like the wild blueberry that comes back stronger than before, we can turn whatever shape our "fire" takes into the accomplishment of brand-new growth. And, like the wild blue berry, we can return after our trauma to the nourishment of ancient wisdom that knows how to thrive. Who knew wild blueberries had so much to say!

BOSSY PANTS

We live in a condo community that features several small lakes. Our second story home overlooks Lake Jasmine, where we can watch a variety of ducks and birds feed, and interact, – it can be quite entertaining. This is what I've observed. There are a number of Mottled Ducks in our neighborhood (Florida is heavily populated with them) that fly between the local lakes to socialize and meet their daily needs. One brown Mottled Duck in particular stands out because of its personality. I've named it "Bossy Pants."

Bossy Pants likes to tell other ducks of its species exactly what to do, and when to do it. It squawks, chases, pecks, and beats its wings at any duck that comes too close, or feeds where it wants to feed. Other ducks fight back but eventually give up because Bossy Pants is persistent. Recently we watched BP reach a new height of bossiness with different results.

There is a fountain in the middle of Lake Jasmine that turns on around 9:00 am. Before it turns on ducks like to perch on the ring and take naps. In the past, groups of ducks have shared the ring quite peacefully. On this particular morning, one duck was sitting on the ring when Bossy Pants landed on the lake. BP looked the situation over, swam straight to the ring that was open, except for one spot, and pecked at the residing duck until it left the ring. No other spot on the ring would do except the one occupied.

All the other Mottled Ducks, who usually hang around on the outskirts of the lake when BP is present, found his behavior unacceptable. They rose up in the air together telling Bossy Pants exactly what they thought, and left. They have, as a group, decided to have nothing to do with BP. It's been ostracized. BP has lost its community and we now see it only by itself. Its obnoxious behavior drove away its support system, and it is now completely ignored by all the other Mottled Ducks.

As I watched this scenario develop, I realized again the importance of community. Building relationships is the cornerstone of community, and that begins with finding connections amongst ourselves. We can connect through our similarities and our differences and, with a sense of appreciation for individual uniqueness, create meaningful relationships that enhance our own lives. What BP doesn't know is solid, strong connections are essential for our health and well-being – even if you're a duck. Who is BP going to huddle with in a storm?

If things get messy in relationship building, and every situation has its up and downs, here are a few suggestions for bridging the gap and keeping community open and healthy. We can set aside time to communicate clearly so misunderstandings don't fester. That means listening without interrupting until it's our turn to speak. It helps to think about what it would be like to be in the other person's shoes and bring compassion into the scenario. That's needed when stress levels are high. It also means being willing to admit when we have made a mistake and apologize.

We build strong ties with expressions of gratitude and treating each other with respect, even when we're disagreeing. What we don't do is sacrifice our personal values to make someone else happy. Our principles are clear in any situation. Reaching out and helping each other, with whatever we have to offer is essential – especially when dealing with a major challenge. Kindness is a miracle worker relieving stress and promoting positive feelings of connectedness and caring.

Support when things get tough builds relationships and community. Marya Axner wrote, "Central to almost every religion is the idea that we should treat our neighbors the way we would like to be treated. If you can keep that in mind, you will most likely succeed in building relationships that you can depend on."[2] Bossy Pants doesn't know this and will be weathering the next storm by itself.

Now is the time to keep in touch so we feel that needed community connection. With that in place we will have the encouragement we need to be our most courageous selves. We will also know beyond a doubt that we're heard, valued, and loved. Bossy Pants is an example of what not to do, which is an important lesson in itself. BP is on its own. I'm glad we have each other and can all huddle together.

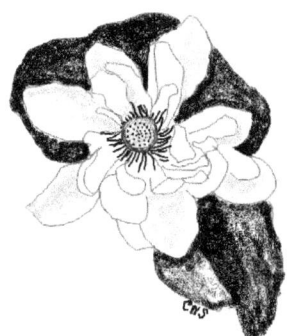

THE LOTUS AND THE MUD

Recently my husband and I went to our local botanical garden when the most water lilies and lotus were blooming. It was a rich time for our senses as we walked the small streams and lakes full of blossoms. We left feeling renewed. I began to ponder how the exquisite lotus comes from a dark, murky place. In its unseen world it draws all the nutrients it can find through its stem to help it mature into a gorgeous lotus flower. It's all the dark, muddy material at the bottom of the pond that feeds its emergence.

To make this more personal, how is our growth fed? Looking back on my life I see my growth was fed by the murky pond of my own inner darkness, the times I struggled most with cancer, surgeries, relationship challenges, job stress, depression and spiritual crisis. I'd like to suggest we all have troubling experiences through the choices we make and their consequences, or the unexpected events that take us by surprise.

All the internal conflicts we live with can feed our seed of potential so the mud of our own life nourishes the personal unfolding of our own version of the beautiful lotus flower. One of the most rewarding things to work toward is our own personal growth. When we reframe our struggles, we know ourself more deeply, let go of what we can't control, accept what is, problem solve more creatively and experience more inner peace. Who wouldn't want more of that?

Here are a few ideas for using our mud to grow. This is not an easy process. It takes time and involves unlearning some old habits and practicing new responses to difficulties. Let's start by facing our fears so they don't stop us before we even get started. Keeping a journal helps us reflect on recent events and gain self-awareness. Paying attention and becoming an active listener helps us understand the people around us. When we cultivate our social skills, we become better at working with a variety of different people. That's personal growth.

More growth occurs when we embrace the truth. It's easy to hide behind unconscious eating, constant activity, or too much alcohol, which blocks the nourishment we need from the truth. Instead let's look at what needs to be seen and let it become part of our blossoming. To help with this we can ground ourself in what nourishes us by breathing deeply, listening to soothing music, being with people who support us, spiritual practices, or enjoying an art form that feeds us most. If we're grounded in the present moment, we can resist the urge to ignore our mud and embrace it instead.

Growth occurs when we organize our home, work and time. Prioritizing helps us work through challenging situations so we can be more flexible and accept change. When we believe in ourself we approach decisions with more confidence because our values and priorities are clear.

If we want to reach our full potential, let's use our transforming mud to get there. We're all developing beautifully when we become our most authentic self. This brings our own precious lotus flower into full bloom. We can thank the dark, murky parts of our life for that.

ANOLE EYES

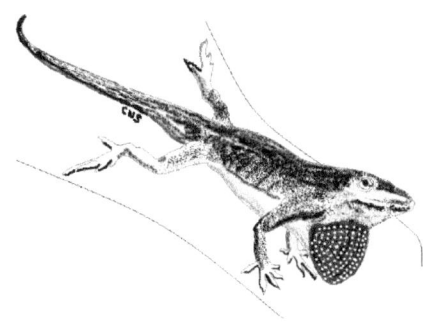

While peacefully journaling
under an ancient oak tree I felt
a presence join me. I was being
watched. The feeling of eyes focused on me was so strong I had to stop
writing and look around. No people were present; no dog was sitting
nearby wagging its tail, rabbits, squirrels, and birds were going about
their morning business. Looking on the ground around me I discovered
my companion. At the base of the tree grew lush ferns and on one fern
frond, partially hidden, was an anole lizard focused completely on me. It
wasn't an intrusive eye, just an inquisitive one.

Quietly I said "Hello, and how are you today?" Its head went back and
forth as though it was looking at me from different angles. Neither of us
moved as we stayed eye to eye, checking each other out. A dialogue
began with me quietly talking but not moving. The anole replied by
nodding its head, periodically puffing up its red throat flag, and moving a
tiny bit closer. After a while I returned to journaling without any further
communication, thinking the anole would go on its way. The next time I
looked the anole was fully revealed, several inches closer, and still
focused on me.

Every time I returned to writing I could feel anole eyes watching me. I
began looking up more often, and always found the anole was right there
focused on me, and a little bit closer. What started out as a questioned
presence, became a pleasant companion and the two of us kept up an
ongoing conversation until it was time for me to leave. We never
touched, but we still connected. It didn't matter that our bodies, life

styles and language were different, we both enjoyed the companionship of eye contact and the safety we felt in slowly getting closer to each other. I had made a friend.

Without eye contact we would not have connected. The same is true with humans. Infants have the ability to look into their caregivers eyes and hold that gaze even if it moves. A.J. Harbinger writes "Eye contact is one of the easiest and most powerful ways to make a person feel recognized, understood and validated."[3] Don't we all want to be understood, validated and recognized? The act of simply holding someone's gaze can create that whether we're beginning a new friendship, or deepening an existing one. Like the anole and I, mutual gazing created pleasure in each other's presence, and a sense of shared closeness.

When we're talking to someone and they are looking around the room instead of looking at us, we know they're not listening. Have you ever had a doctor do that to you? They do need to type information into their computers when they're working with us, but if they aren't taking time to look us in the eye, especially when we're asking questions, or expressing a concern, we're in the wrong place. It's time for a different doctor.

Often, we can tell how a person is feeling by looking in their eyes. Sometimes we don't even need to ask them how they are, we can see the excitement, joy, sadness, pain and every other emotion without a word being said. Then we can offer support, encouragement, laughter, help or hugs as needed. It's a meaningful gift to meet eye to eye. If looking at an anole lizard can bring an animal and human closer, think how much more we can enrich our daily relationships connecting person to person through the power of eye contact. I'm going to see what more I can learn about myself and others as I practice this connecting skill. Anyone care to join me?

INSIDE THE CHRYSALIS

On Sunday we pick up The New York Times Newspaper from my sister and enjoy a leisurely amble through its pages. Included in each edition is

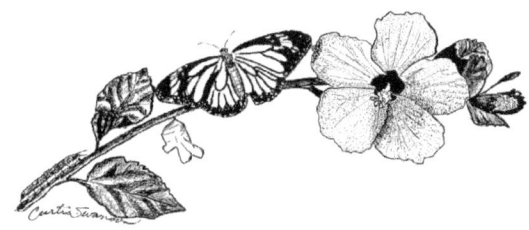

The New York Times Magazine which features timely articles. I was instantly attracted to an article titled "The Truth About Cocoons" by Sam Anderson.[4] Those of you who know me know that my favorite illustration of transformation is the caterpillar to butterfly story. Life is rich with times to draw inside, process change, and reemerge with new wings.

What struck me about the article was its emphasis on what happens inside the cocoon, which in the case of a butterfly is actually a chrysalis. Like the author, I realized that I had spent most of my time thinking about the before and after, and very little time thinking about what happens during the confinement. In the darkness, during the waiting, the caterpillar slowly disintegrates until it is caterpillar soup, with only a couple of organs left to help start the rebuilding process. In Sam Anderson's words, "Only after this near-total self-annihilation can the new growth begin." The butterfly comes only after the total meltdown of the modest caterpillar.

Any crisis can offer the opportunity to go within to rethink everything before reemerging. It could be a financial set back, death of a loved one, depression, diagnosis of a life-threatening illness (cancer did this for me), or the ending of a long relationship. During COVID it was amazing to see how the world did stop, together we went inside, and together we stayed home. Our familiar structures changed. The inside of the chrysalis is a mirror for us as we look at it both from a personal view, and as a society.

The beauty in the mess is that a breakdown always precedes a rebuilding. Sam Anderson writes, "The metamorphoses are happening mostly in private, all over the place, in billions of individual pods – acts of internal self-destruction and rebuilding, subtle shifts and whole revolutions." There are seeds of transformation in the scary, uncomfortable, dark, mushy soup. Individually we are not the same and collectively we are asking for change. There will always be voices of discord, and malcontents who are never satisfied. They do not represent the majority who are willing to embrace the uncomfortable place of doing life differently, and commit to improving their lives and the lives of others.

Inner transformation comes from letting go of everything that no longer serves us; uncaring doctors, abusive relationships, negative attitudes, limiting beliefs, harmful habits. There's an alchemy that takes place that involves the death of the old and the birth of the new. The alchemy involves loving ourselves enough to accept our imperfections, treating ourselves with respect, and practicing self-compassion. Little by little, every small effort builds on the next until something magnificent is created. For the butterfly chrysalis, the slow assembly of the body, head, and wings make the butterfly happen.

We don't awaken when we are comfortable; we awaken when we're uncomfortable. Yes, transformation is hard and scary, and at times we'll want to stop, but it is the most rewarding work we will ever do. Transformation happens when we realize no one is responsible for our lives but ourselves. It happens when we take responsibility for how we act and react. It happens when we make decisions based on what we truly desire, and not on what someone else wants for us. It happens when we look for positive ways to use life's opportunities, and when we support equality and peaceful solutions. It happens when we love unconditionally.

Individually we are looking out a hole in our chrysalises bringing our changes within, to the changes without. Already we are seeing with new eyes as we hold the potential of soaring with new wings. Marianne Williamson writes, "Personal transformation can and does have global effects. As we go, so goes the world, for the world is us. The revolution that will save the world is ultimately a personal one."[5] We're learning what we need to inside the chrysalis, and the results will show.

Dear people who are willing to break down to come together in a new way, you are some of the most transformed. You are the colorful butterflies that inspire others because you know all about being inside the chrysalis. Thank you to those who share their journey and show their beautiful selves! This is one experience none of us want to miss.

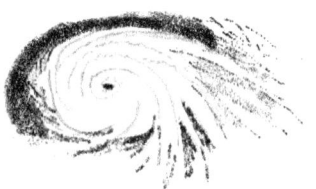

HURRICANE IRMA'S ANGELS

How quiet and peaceful the weather is now compared to when Hurricane Irma was howling and beating horizontal rain against our windows. It was an intense, noisy, fascinating, unforgettable and scary experience! My sister stayed with us in our home here in Vero Beach and, as the storm progressed, I kept thinking how difficult it would be to be alone during this kind of weather experience. There was comfort in our togetherness as we felt our building vibrate, saw gutters come down,

11

shingles lift off a portion of a neighbor's roof and trees fall. But it could have been so much worse!

As the hurricane moved north and we all began coming out of our homes, acts of kindness became abundant, as though angels were working in concert to meet the many needs left in Irma's wake. I am so deeply moved by our own experience and the stories told to me by others, that I wanted to share some of them with you.

My sister lives in a neighborhood of elders who needed help putting storm shutters up as Irma approached. The people hired to do the job left a number of homes undone. When the young woman who cleans my sister's house heard this, she determined to take care of the problem. On her own time Saturday, she and a muscular male friend arrived and took care of shuttering all the homes she works in every week and let all the residents (who had been ordered to evacuate) know there was no need to worry - their windows were protected.

My hair stylist shared how all the young people in her neighborhood put storm shutters up for their elderly residents. They made sure everyone had food which included inviting those living by themselves to join the family for dinner. As soon as a need was known help was provided.

After the hurricane my sister and I were sitting on our front porch when three women from our neighborhood drove by and asked how we were doing. We responded with assurances that we were fine but the power was off. Then they asked us if we needed anything and we lightly said yes, we need ice, thinking of our slowly warming refrigerator. An hour later the same three women came to our front door with two large bags of ice (How did they find this when every store seemed to be out?) that saved the food in our refrigerator. They would not let me reimburse them insisting it was a gift. I told them they were Irma Angels.

A utility pole came down in the yard of my chiropractor requiring a crew of workers and several hours of hard work. His wife fired up their grill and made everyone hamburgers along with a steady flow of cold drinks. The workers were very grateful for the break and the food!

Walking into a store I was hailed by one of the employees I often see when shopping. This was Friday and she was still out of power. Every night people with restored power offered her a place to stay so she could get a good night's rest. Her niece, wanting to help her aunt, stopped where several power trucks were parked and talked to one of the crew. She explained where her aunt lived and asked why her aunt didn't have power yet. The man she was talking to said they had serviced that area but he would personally look into what happened and take care of it himself. And he did.

A family trying to return home was caught needing gas. The gas station was waiting for a delivery so cars were hopefully lined up. The family was exhausted, travel weary, hungry and looking for a place to spend the night. A man, who had gas in his car and had come to the station for something else, saw how weary and stressed the family was. Approaching them he introduced himself and quickly realized what they needed. He and his wife offered the family a small vacation house they had nearby that had sustained no damage from the storm and still had power. The family could spend a night or two there while waiting for gas. The man and his wife took the family out to dinner and then to their vacation house which lifted everyone's spirits. Natural disasters can bring out the best in people.

There are so many more stories to tell! Today's local newspaper has more inspiring accounts of people reaching out to others with kindness, compassion, and generosity. Sometimes angels have familiar faces and sometimes they come as complete strangers, but the level of giving that Irma has stimulated can make all of us proud of the community and county we live in. Other areas hit harder will need long term help, but those needs will also be met. This quote from Adyashanti says it all, "Grace is all around us, if we only have the eyes to see it."[6]

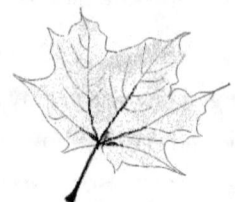

LET'S TURN OVER A NEW LEAF

After living many years in northern states where seasonal change is more dramatic, I now enjoy the subtle seasonal changes of Florida. But northern autumn colors have always been my favorite, and I still relish taking fall internet color tours. In Michigan, when our two children were very young we used to collect bright leaves, dip them in wax, and use them for table decorations. We turned leaves over frequently, looking at all the color combinations. That memory reminded me of the expression "turning over a new leaf."

So, I googled the expression "turning over a new leaf" and learned something new. This expression started in the 16th century and did not refer to tree leaves, but instead to book pages. The expression meant turning over the present page and leaving the past behind for a fresh start on a new page. This expression invites changing course and rethinking choices for a new beginning.

As the leaves change color, we too can release ourselves from staying the same by turning over a new personal leaf. We can challenge ourselves to grow into healthier behaviors and learn from every experience, no matter how uncomfortable. The best way to do this is to be open to change. Change can feel intimidating because it takes us out of our comfort zone, especially when it involves our health, relationships, or financial stability. But to move forward for any fresh start, we need to embrace change.

We can turn over a new leaf in self-care by being selfish in the very best way. This means checking our decision-making to see if what we're doing is benefiting others more than ourselves. If we're giving ourselves away to everyone else, we need to take back control of our life. This is the time to remind ourselves that we're not able to take care of anyone else until we've taken care of ourselves first.

Another helpful new leaf is letting go of what is no longer working in our life. Letting go of a long-term relationship can be difficult because we're heavily invested in this person, but if this relationship is no longer healthy, it's polluting our life. We need to release it, step forward, and leave it in the past. During a serious illness we may discover we need to change our medical facility, doctor, or treatment plan. We may need to redo our budget to accommodate changing circumstances. Eckhart Tolle writes, "Sometimes letting things go is an act of far greater power than defending or hanging on."[7]

Let's develop a new attitude about what we call failure, and celebrate it instead of criticizing ourselves. It's easy to applaud achievements, but valuable lessons lie in our blunders. Failure is a teacher showing us what we don't want. Eckhart Tolle writes, "It is through the mistakes that the greatest learning happens on an inner level."[8]

Let's turn over a new leaf on negative thoughts and liberate ourselves from them especially if they are about our bodies. If we leave behind the judgements about too-big thighs or flabby arms and love ourselves just as we are, we will discover our own unique beauty. All we need is to be open to positive change. Let's turn over a new page in our personal book and begin to implement those needed changes that have been percolating in the back of our minds. This is the perfect time for turning over a new leaf.

MOUNTAIN WILDERNESS

There is a beautiful story in Howard Thurman's "Meditations of the Heart"[9] that describes his unique climbing experience with a different kind of mountain wilderness. The following is his story in my words.

Howard climbed until he was above the timber line and noticed how the forest had abruptly stopped, as though there was an invisible barrier. Above the tree line was a rocky bareness punctuated with patches of snow, strong winds, and what looked like small clusters of evergreen bushes. He wondered how anything could survive and grow in this hostile environment. The greens were not lush, but they were alive and strong.

Howard looked more closely and noticed that the plant needles were a perfect match to the trees further down the mountain. As he continued to study them, he thought they resembled branches from the trees. In amazement he realized they were tree branches hugging the ground like vines as they followed the shape of their terrain. Because of the harsh landscape they could not grow upright, but that did not keep them from growing. What looked like stunted shrubs were actually rows of growing tree branches.

Howard marveled at the determined struggle that had produced this unusual phenomenon. It felt as though he could hear the trees saying that, although they could not reach for the heavens as they normally would, they did not want to die. They carefully surveyed what they had to work with and put together a way to experience growth and development, despite the harsh living conditions. They survived where nothing else could, knowing the only way to thrive was to change. In the end, the branches did not look like the other trees, but instead of giving up, they fully used every resource available to answer life with life. They embraced what they had, and affirmed a universe that sustains and celebrates life in all its forms. This is where Howard's acute observations and story ends.

Courageous people this is exactly what we do. When we're in that desolate place of drastic change, we may no longer be able to do and be what we once were. How we look and what we do may change. We use all our resources to keep ourselves encouraged as we navigate new ways to fully live within our environment. Challenged to our core, we still find a way to thrive.

We are determined and strong because we are linked together as branches from the same tree. We know how to change what needs changing to survive. Together we support each other through every harsh wind and trying moment of our mountain wilderness. We know already what Howard Thurman discovered – together we can face life's toughest challenges, and transform them into inner growth and wisdom. Eckhart Tolle writes, "The key to transformation is to make friends with this moment. What form it takes doesn't matter. Say yes to it. Allow it. Be with it."[10]

No matter where you are in your wilderness experience, know you are in a sacred place. Susan Vreeland writes it beautifully in this quote, "No matter where life takes you, the place you stand at any moment is holy ground. Love hard, and love wide and love long and you will find the goodness in it."[11]

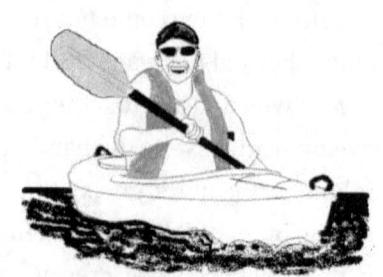

NURTURING THROUGH NATURE

Whether it's walking through the surf
on the beach, sitting under a tree
watching the sun dance on the leaves, or for me, kayaking the Indian
River Lagoon, being outdoors nurtures our body, mind and spirit. If we're
confined indoors, turning off our digital gadgets, and sitting by a window
that gives a view of the sky, trees, and flowering plants, will still give a
boost to our brains and bodies. Bringing green or flowering plants
indoors will also improve our overall sense of well-being.

Nature is a calming elixir available to us whenever we choose to step
outside, or bring it indoors. David Gessner wrote in National Geographic,
"Science is proving what we've always known intuitively: nature does
good things for the human brain — it makes us healthier, happier, and
smarter."[12] With time in nature our brains command center can dial
down and rest, enhancing peace, empathy, and connectivity.

For me, nature has always been an essential element to my well-being. It
is my therapist when I need to destress, my inspiration when I need a
vitality boost, and a comfort when I need to work through loss. In nature
I feel a connection with something greater than myself, and a bond with
other life forms. This is deeply nurturing.

During any time of stress, we can use a dose of "forest bathing," which is
widely done in Japan. This is a leisurely walk through a forest, park, or
bamboo grove, taking in the atmosphere of the trees around us. This
lowers both pulse rate and blood pressure, decreases the stress hormone
cortisol, and increases the immune function. Spending time with trees

also helps reduce inflammation in our bodies. Inflammation is behind many of our illnesses so this is encouraging news.

Author Allison Dienstman wrote, "10 Unexpected Benefits of Spending Time in Nature"[13] which featured the results of studies on this topic. Here are some of the things she learned. From the University of Michigan came a study that revealed that regular walking enhanced memory retention. Now that's one I can use! As little as five minutes a day outside can help reduce stress, and only 20 minutes of sunshine a day will increase levels of Vitamin D, which strengthens bones, and helps the body resist disease. Time in natural light improves our sleep pattern, strengthens our immune system and boosts our mood.

Too much time on our various screens can damage our eye sight, but time outdoors supports our vision. All the colors, shapes, smells, and textures found in nature are inspiring, and this boosts our creativity. John P. Milton writes, "Today, our modern world is filled with high-tech wonders. When we leave these tensions for a while to cultivate our natural wholeness in the wild, we are renewed with the fresh vitality and spirit of Nature. New pathways open for living in harmony with our communities and the Earth. We discover deep inspiration to help transform our lifestyles and our culture toward harmony and balance."[14]

Nurturing through nature develops us spiritually because we clear our minds of clutter as we take time to see sun sparkles on the water, feel the breeze on our skin, or watch the tiny Anole lizard running in front of us. When we're quietly relaxed outdoors, our brain waves become like the brain waves experienced in meditation, so we feel refreshed, renewed, and connected to our Higher Power.

Nature is a meaningful metaphor for resiliency. When a forest fire happens, the forest regrows and regenerates. It will always recover, heal, and begin again, which is symbolic of how we can overcome our difficult experiences. A river can remind us to go with the flow, while a bird song is an invitation to stay in the moment. We aren't just observers of nature, we are a part of nature. It is instinctive for us to take the steps needed to nourish ourselves because we are a harmonious part of the whole. Let's make spending more time in nature a habit, and, when life circumstances keep us indoors, let's bring nature indoors by taking care of a plant, purchasing an orchid, or bringing inside a shell or rock that speaks to us. We can tour gardens on line. Nurturing through nature doesn't cost us anything but a little time, and the payback is tremendous. There's nothing to lose and much to gain. Maybe I'll see you on my next walk.

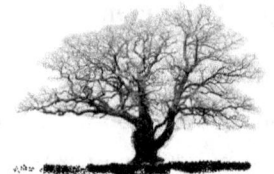

STILLNESS UNDER THE ANCIENT OAK

The ancient oak tree was fascinating! Locals think the elderly tree is at least 250 years old. It has a huge trunk base from which nine large separate trunks emerged. I kept walking around the tree to make sure I was counting correctly, and yes, nine large trunks came out of the base. The towering branches formed an umbrella shape around the spacious lawn and long strands of moss danced in the wind. Two metal chains held an old fashioned, double seater, wood slat swing from a lower branch. The invitation to sit within the world of this tree was irresistible. Everything else was let go as I sat in the swing and gently swayed myself into stillness.

It was as though the oak tree held a world of its own under its canopy. Two doves sat on a lower branch cooing and surveying their realm, while Anole lizards sunned themselves on large fern fronds at the base of the tree, flashing their red throat flags. A cicada choir ebbed and flowed sounding like a group of rusty doors. Mocking birds called to each other while they ignored squirrels energetically running across branches. A variety of butterflies flew by on their way to a nearby bush full of orange blossoms. Two cardinals perched on branches long enough to evaluate the area for breakfast and select a grassy place worth investigating. Ants and insects were busy with their day's work. A variety of different colored lichen grew along the branches, as well as air plants, and blooming wild orchids. This is the kind of abundance in nature that I notice only when I'm still. It's the beauty of small things that I miss when I'm rushing to my next destination or project.

Often stillness is viewed as being unproductive, but in reality stillness can be our greatest allay. In stillness we renew ourselves and our perspective, so balance is maintained. In stillness new beginnings emerge and clarity is gained. Stillness is where priorities are determined and creativity is birthed. It is where new beginnings emerge, love is understood, and we can come home to our true peaceful selves. Stillness offers us an opportunity for reflection, and provides relief from thoughts of trying to control what could or should be happening. It's the best therapy for tension and anxiety because it enhances inner peace.

Eckhart Tolle says in his book **Stillness Speaks**, "The moment you become aware of a plant's emanation of stillness and peace, that plant becomes your teacher."[15] My teacher was the ancient oak tree that showed me how many forms of life can live in harmony, how thinking too much about the future can mask the beauty of this moment, how focusing on what I love brings me joy, how patience with change will clarify the gift it's bringing. And, like the ancient oak, I can accept whatever comes, acknowledge its presence, and let it pass through me. Tree branches don't grab and hold onto anything, but let whatever storm is passing travel through and be released. What a healthy way to handle life's storms.

21

Of course, to be still we need to slow down. Author Yo Bronwyn writes, "Please don't feel guilty about slowing down. Don't regret a day, a month, or a year in a quiet state of not doing. Doing is not your only purpose. Feeling, opening, receiving, contemplating, listening deeply, seeing deeply – these quiet (non)acts of stillness also have their purpose."[16] Stillness nourishes us so more inner resources are available when action is needed.

While I was under the tree there were several noisy interruptions from grounds keepers. I noticed that with each interruption my focus changed temporarily. That was followed by the opportunity to go right back to stillness so, my choice determined what I focused on, and what I focused on determined my personal nourishment. That's worth remembering. We don't need to be under a tree to experience stillness. We can select our own stillness place and experience the gifts that will bring.

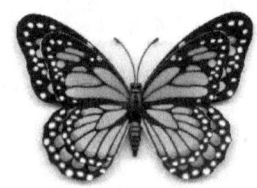

THE ORANGE BUTTERFLY

Following the sandy path led me through tall tropical trees hung with moss, flowering bushes, graceful ferns, low blooming wild flowers, and vines that climbed whatever was in their path. Even though I wasn't far from civilization I enjoyed the feeling of being in a jungle. In the middle of this setting an orange butterfly caught my attention. Standing still I watched it navigate the surrounding greenery until it selected the perfect place to land. It chose a tall narrow leaf to settle on and a beautiful lesson unfolded.

Arranging itself with wings wide open, the butterfly tried to maintain its balance while the wind gave it a challenge. Its first position kept it unbalanced so, with wings still open, it rearranged itself. The wind now upset the orange wings even more. The third position involved completely folding up its wings and placing itself against the wind. It was almost blown off the tall leaf. The fourth position involved keeping its wings folded and facing into the wind. This produced no wind resistance and the desired balance was achieved. The butterfly settled into a time of rest.

As I watched this process, I was struck by the effort the butterfly had put into its endeavor for balance, and how facing into the wind was the only way to find it. It reminded me of myself and how I was handling the winds of change in my life. Like the orange butterfly, I had been experimenting with different approaches, but was not achieving the desired outcome. My wind has been a multitude of changes that revealed the need to do life differently. What worked in the past was no longer appropriate. I needed to stop fighting against the wind which always makes life more difficult than it needs to be. Only recently have I finally faced into the wind and felt the relief of letting go of struggle.

Watching the orange butterfly also reminded me of how shore birds stand facing into the wind when a storm is coming. Other birds line up facing the same direction on a power line. If the wind shifts the birds will change their position so they are always facing into the wind – facing into the challenge. Rev. Margret A. O'Neall writes, "We can face into the wind, face into the future, and so we are prepared to move forward, to move into the winds of change, embracing the future in whatever way we will."[17]

Whether we are moving into a new relationship, addressing a serious health issue, changing jobs, creating a healthy home, or committing to a new activity, change will ask us to look at life differently. When we stand in our strength facing into the wind, we can accept what is happening with the wisdom of previous experience and the gift of balance. Like the birds, we have companions for facing our challenges and weathering the storm. Like the orange butterfly we can rest easy in the winds of change. What a relief to let go of struggle and embrace balance while making needed changes.

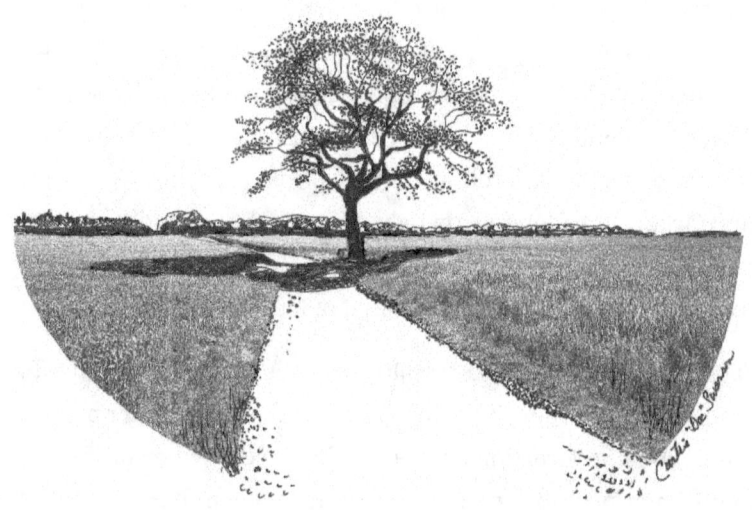

Chapter 2 – Inspiration

YOU RAISE ME UP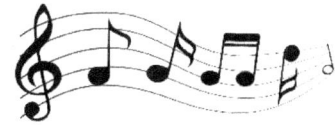

"You Raise Me Up" is the title of a song with lyrics by Irish songwriter Brendan Graham.[1] The song took its time to come to America, but when it did, interpretations by artists like Josh Groban, touched an emotional chord of appreciation. Here are the words to the chorus:

You raise me up, so I can stand on mountains

You raise me up to walk on stormy seas

I am strong when I am on your shoulders

You raise me up: To more than I can be.

We are stronger and more powerful together. We overcome challenges well together. Together we can accomplish more than we can individually. When we support each other, we are at our very best. We do this for each other, and our Higher Power does this for us every day.

As human beings we are wired for nurturing relationships, so it's difficult to watch all the negativity from our media programing. Destructive behavior injures us all, but the opposite is also true: When we empower, support, and encourage each other, we diffuse the negative and raise the vibrational frequencies of ourselves and everyone around us. As Robert Ingersoll writes, "We rise by lifting others."[2]

Recently my husband and I had a conversation about all the times we have lifted each other up during our marriage so we could accomplish something significant that would not have otherwise happened. We only did these things because we took turns standing on each other's shoulders and supporting each other through stormy seas.

It's a privilege to enjoy the companionship of people we love, so here are a few ideas about how we can raise each other up. We lift each other up when we live in our own incredible worth without having to put someone else down. Treating each other with kindness and compassion builds love and support for everyone around us.

Raising up happens when we treat people with respect that is shared. However, this means having zero tolerance for abusive talk, gossip, or bullying. We remove our self from media that specializes in spreading fear and "hearing" the people who trash-talk. Thinking before we speak means our words come from a thoughtful place, and we honor any confidence that is shared so it goes no further.

Verbally sharing and applauding each other's successes lifts everyone involved. Encouraging words are an expression of presence and sincerity. "Lifters" love to share knowledge in the form of helpful articles, books, or tools on the web when it offers an inspiring discovery, new learning, or an appropriate application to our life.

We build each other up when we stay humble, no matter how much we accomplish. When we feel secure, we don't need to brag, and everyone around us is treated with equality. We're positive in a way that is contagious because we're open to the benefits of differences and the potential in change.

Lifting up requires taking the time to understand the whole story and being quick to offer forgiveness. Understanding means being a careful listener, accepting what is being shared and answering when asked without judging. Raising up also needs patience. Joyce Meyer writes, "Patience is not simply the ability to wait — it's how we behave while we're waiting."[3]

We raise each other highest when we love. The attributes of love bring out the best in all of us because love is not easily angered, is not self-seeking; it's kind, patient, hopeful, perseveres, protects, respects, and honors truth. Those are all ingredients for thriving. Jim Stovall writes, "You need to be aware of what others are doing, applaud their efforts, acknowledge their successes, and encourage them in their pursuits. When we all help one another, everybody wins."[4] Together we can walk this stormy sea. Together we can stand on each other's shoulders and be strong. Together we are so much more than we can be alone

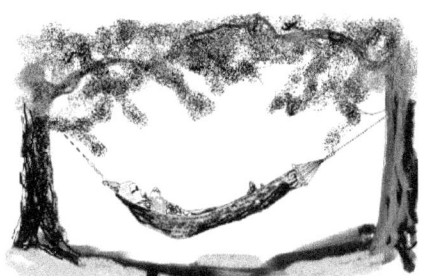

CULTIVATING CONTENTMENT

Contentment is more than a moment of passing appreciation, it's a way of life, a way of being. It's that place deep inside where our minds and hearts rest because we're at ease with who we are and what we have. Contentment does not mean overlooking what is painful or difficult, but instead letting go of the struggle and focusing on the gifts that always accompany a challenge. In the midst of heartache, mindfulness and contentment widen our field of awareness enabling us to embrace what's difficult, instead of being overwhelmed by it. This gives us the vision to see all the nourishing aspects of this moment.

Contentment is a powerful choice, and since we are the curators of our own contentment, let's think about how to cultivate this. Doris Mortman wrote, "Until you make peace with who you are, you will never be content with what you have."[5] Making peace begins with accepting who we are and loving ourself with the same deep commitment that we give

27

to others. We show ourself kindness, become our own best friend, and acknowledge that we're not in competition with anyone else. We avoid harsh judgements, forgive ourself when needed and learn from our mistakes.

Mayo Clinic writes that science tells us only a small portion of our contentedness comes from circumstances. Most of it comes from our personal thoughts and behaviors, and those can be changed. Contented people seem to know this gift comes from the sum of their life choices. According to Mayo Clinic Staff, the pillars for those choices are - investing in relationships, appreciating what we have, having a positive outlook, having a sense of purpose and living in the moment.

Recognizing when we have enough is another way to cultivate contentment. Things take time and energy to maintain, so passing on what we don't need simplifies life and feels freeing. My husband and I have discovered that the older we get, the less we need. This leaves more time for things we enjoy and many of these are completely free such as: reading poetry to each other, walking on the beach, cooking a favorite meal together, watching ducks and birds come and go on the lake, and "face time" with family. Contentment can come from life's little pleasures.

Gratitude nourishes contentment because it promotes a sense of wonder and appreciation for life. Both life's large and small events deserve gratitude so I'm grateful for the first hot drink of the morning, fresh sheets on the bed, the orchid blooming in the living room, the wind on my face, and the driver who lets me into a crowded lane of traffic. Thanking someone who's shown us kindness or supported us through a hard time uplifts both the person giving thanks, and the receiver. Gratitude is a counterpoint that gently focuses our attention on everything we have to be thankful for, instead of letting our minds get stuck in what we feel is lacking in our life.

Our contentment is increased when we make time to be quiet. Some people do this by meditating, which stimulates the part of the brain that makes us feel good. Meditation can take different forms such as praying, listening to nature, or walking through a park. The purpose of quiet time is to connect with our inner guidance so we're listening to our heart. This connection leads to an inner peace and calmness that heals and strengthens us, so stress and anxiety are reduced.

We cultivate contentment when we do what we love, take time to have fun, stay in the moment and accept the things we can't change. Since all of this is a matter of choice, we hold the key to open contentment. Consider this an open invitation to increasing the nourishing aspects of our life. Let's choose to be at ease with who we are and what we have so we can deepen our daily contentment.

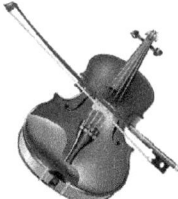

DISGUISED OPPORTUNITIES

When Tyler Butler-Figueroa was 4 ½ years old he was diagnosed with leukemia. He came close to dying several times during his long treatment. When he was well enough to go to school, he was bullied for having no hair, and a student rumor was spread that his cancer was contagious so everyone stayed away from him. He became discouraged and wanted to give up on everything. One day he noticed a school flyer about an after-school program for kids who wanted to learn to play an instrument. A violin caught his eye and he asked to try the program.

Tyler discovered he could pour all his emotions into the violin, and slowly his feelings evolved from depression to joy as he experienced the pleasure of expressing his new found love of life. Soon he was combining music and dance steps with playful enthusiasm. His musical talent brought him to America's Got Talent at age eleven where he qualified for the finals. He brought the house down with his performance, and the judges thanked him for taking something intensely difficult and turning it into inspiring music and dance. Tyler's comment was, "I used to be the kid with cancer, now I'm the kid who plays violin."[6]

At age eighteen, Mandy Harvey lost her hearing because of a connective tissue disorder. She had been singing since age four and her dream was to sing professionally, but her vocal training stopped when she became deaf. Her first reaction was to give up in discouragement. After a year she began carefully experimenting to see if there was another way she could still feel and hear music. Using muscle memory and vibrations, she slowly began to reconnect with her treasured notes.

Then she composed her own song titled "Try."[7] It was her way of saying she wanted to do more with her life than give up, so she took the word "try" as her word for doing what she wanted to do with her life, despite her impairment. At age twenty-one she was a contestant on AGT and, as she stood on the platform in her stocking feet, (so she could feel the vibrations) playing her guitar and singing, she brought the judges to tears with the quality and inspiring message of her music. She qualified for finals.

John Fitzgerald Kennedy wrote, "When written in Chinese, the word "crisis" is composed of two characters – one represents danger, the other represents opportunity."[8] We have all experienced changes in our lives that have challenged us to our very core. When those troubling, unwanted experiences take us out of our comfort zone, we can choose to give up, or we can optimize our new opportunity.

Here are a few suggestions for moving from challenge to opportunity. What we focus on makes all the difference. If we focus on fear and anxiety, we will create a sense of despair that will leave us feeling powerless. Deliberately changing our focus to exploring opportunities inherent in a crisis will move us into a state of empowerment, strength, and action, as seen in the stories of Tyler and Mandy.

Let's be honest with ourselves and identify our true feelings. Embracing our discouragement or sadness is part of being true to ourselves, and makes it easier to enter into the transformational process. Next, we need to stop resisting unwanted change. This calls for a perspective that acknowledges that somewhere in the big picture is a gift waiting to be unwrapped. Mary Roberts Rinehart writes, "Every crucial experience can be regarded as a setback, or the start of a wonderful new adventure, it depends on your perspective."[9]

Another way to find the disguised opportunity is to be open and ready to move on from the point of crisis. This willingness to move on will help keep us from getting stuck. We need to release our hold on loss before we can embrace our relationship with opportunity. Our curiosity can help us embrace new ideas which can lead to reflecting on how we would like to do things differently. Obstacles can present us with open time we didn't have before so we can explore new skills, or complete projects that have been waiting. During COVID I tackled all kinds of projects around our home that had been on hold. Bernice Johnson Reagon [10]writes, "Life's challenges are not supposed to paralyze you, they're supposed to help you discover who you are." That's exactly what Tyler and Mandy did. Let's take life's challenges and look for every opportunity offered, no matter how disguised they may be. Each one is a gift.

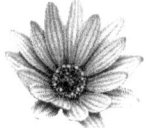

EVERYDAY BLISS

Often bliss is associated with a state of euphoria that is infrequently experienced because it depends on sensational circumstances. Bliss doesn't have anything to do with circumstances because it is an inner state of being that is nourished by listening to the voice of our heart. Our heart's voice leads us to love. It's through love that we connect to everyday bliss.

Since conception begins in a moment of ecstasy, bliss is our origin. This origin is always waiting to be tapped into and expressed as our most natural state of unconditional love. Sometimes we disconnect from this when others hurt or betray us, or we betray ourself. We can choose what to do with our emotional wounds and unwanted baggage by deciding to let go of the grievances. The power of forgiveness will lead to healing and reconnecting to the bliss of our origin.

It's comforting to know that everyday bliss does not depend on getting the dream job, finding the perfect mate, or having a fantastic vacation. It resides inside each of us and there are things we can do to help cultivate it. It starts by being more loving to first ourself and then to others. If we have a problem, we can ask ourself how to bring love into the situation. When we make a mistake (and we all do), rather than criticizing ourself let's listen to our heart's voice and invite love in to release the tension and restore perspective.

Bliss blooms when we are kind to ourself and others – even when they are rude. What!? When we shift our fucus from rude people to being kind, we are choosing to respond rather than react. When we cultivate love we let go of judgement, fear, shame, and anger and return to everyday bliss. Everyday bliss develops when we practice compassion, respect our own needs and give as generously as our resources allow. It also happens when we're open minded and realize our connectedness with everything. We are not a separate being.

Here are a few clues to knowing we are experiencing everyday bliss. We feel gratitude just to be alive and throughout the day we notice little things that give us pleasure. There are frequent experiences of synchronicity and we can see how life is working for us – not against us. We feel energetic, creative, and completely alive. There is a deep sense of purpose and meaning along with the knowledge that we're contributing to the collective good. Deeper bonds with others are developed. The heart's voice is listened to and love is the lens through which all life is seen. Identify with any of these and we're on our way.

Author Sean Meshorer wrote, "Bliss is like a white light. Just as pure light is the totality of all color, bliss is the conglomeration of all positive qualities. When seen through the prism of spiritual awareness, the subcomponents are joy, unconditional love, inner peace, power, connectedness, awe, and wisdom. Bliss cannot be attained, really. The soul simply realizes that bliss simply is. It is what remains after everything external and fleeting disappears."[11]

Bliss is love because it includes all states and emotions just the way white includes all color. We are wrapped in everyday bliss when we love ourself and listen to the voice of our heart. Let's all connect with the beautiful qualities of everyday bliss that deepens the love that each day holds. Love is the key – bliss is the result.

EVERYDAY SUCCESS

Our American culture defines success in terms of power, prestige, and money, which deprives the term of its greater meaning. Ralph Waldo Emerson writes this definition of success, "To laugh often and much; to win the respect of intelligent people and the affection of children; to leave the world a better place; to know that even one life has breathed easier because you have lived. This is to have succeeded."[12]

We can't all be poet laureates, or win a Nobel Peace Prize. We may not have invented the technology tool that connects us with people all over the world, but when we do what we can, and reach out to each other, we enrich the lives of everyone around us, often more than we know. And if it's hard for us to notice or acknowledge our own areas of success, let's use this as a reminder of the difference we can make.

Those of us who have dealt with cancer know there are days that are so difficult that our first thought is to shut down. However, when we choose a treatment plan that is right for us, we are succeeding. When we complete another round of chemo or radiation, laugh at our bald head, get out of bed for a few minutes, or continue drug therapy, we are succeeding. Even when, after careful evaluation, we make the hard choice to stop treatment, we are still working in our best interest and therefore succeeding. When we choose even a minor change towards healthy eating, do our stretching exercises, and create a positive environment around us that nurtures others, we have reason to feel proud of our success. When we practice focused introspection to better know ourselves, and make meditation a priority, we reap the benefits of knowing this is happening for us, not to us. Our inner peace makes the world a more peaceful place. These are all steps to creating a peaceful and successful life, even in the middle of cancer.

Everyday success is also found in forgiving others, instead of holding a grudge, so peace of mind can ripple back into the world. Forgiving ourselves and letting go of the past can be even harder. If we can love ourselves enough to give ourselves a break, our ability to love others is enhanced and love ripples into the world. When we avoid the urge to dominate a conversation and choose to listen so someone can find their own way, compassion ripples into the world. When we take time to express appreciation for someone's positive efforts that might go unnoticed, gratitude and confidence ripples into the world. And when we own a mistake and use it as a point of growth, forgiveness and maturity ripple into the world.

Joe Girard wrote, "The elevator to success is out of order. You'll have to use the stairs. . . .one step at a time."[13] That is how everyday success works. Helping someone who you know can't offer anything in return is a step. Finding pleasure in your work or, in my case, putting my heart into my writing is another step. When we enjoy ourselves, even though our "to do lists" aren't finished, we're still stepping into everyday success because enjoyment is success. Lists are meant to be guidelines, not unbendable chores. Keeping an open mind and learning from someone else creates new possibilities for loving relationships. Any time we create art, music, poetry, storytelling, jewelry or games with heart and positive intention, we release love into the world.

Sometimes everyday success is pulling away from activity and having a quiet, nurturing cup of your favorite beverage in the middle of the day, and sometimes it is walking away from a person or situation that is toxic for us. If we know what matters to us and consistently take daily steps to fill our lives with meaning, we will live with the kind of passion and purpose that inspires us, as well as the people around us. This is just a small beginning of what everyday success looks like, but it's enough to start us thinking. Let's take a closer look at our days – I think you will find they are full of everyday success that ripples quiet inspiration to those around you.

FINDING BEAUTY

It is both profound and uplifting to see beauty in people and the world around us. If our definition of beauty is narrow, we might agree with Miss Piggy from The Muppets who says, "Beauty is in the eye of the beholder and it may be necessary from time to time to give a stupid or misinformed beholder a black eye."[14] Miss Piggy was very good at giving black eyes, especially when her physical appearance was criticized. However, if we are willing to expand our definition of beauty beyond physical beauty, or what is overtly beautiful to others, we improve the quality of our lives. When we look deeper and more meaningfully at people, nature, animals, art, music, and all the inanimate things in our life, we discover more beauty that feeds our contentment and happiness.

Beauty brings transformation the way a smile transforms a face. And every face is its own landscape, quietly vibrant with life's experiences. I think the most beautiful faces are seen on people who know they are loved, because love changes how we see ourselves and others. Love lights us from within, and when people are lit from within, that light spreads beauty the way one candle lit a full sanctuary of candles at the Christmas Eve service we attended. No one's light is diminished by sharing it with another.

Blaise Pascal said, "In difficult times you should always carry something beautiful in your mind."[15] For those times when life seems all struggle and endurance, our heart may feel hurt and broken. It may be difficult to see beauty when we feel broken by a health crisis, the loss of a loved one, or the end of financial security. When we're in that place we may identify with what Anna White writes, "Maybe it's not about having a beautiful day, but finding beautiful moments. Maybe a whole day is just too much to ask. I could choose to believe that in every day, in all things, no matter how dark and ugly, there are shards of beauty if I look for them."[16]

Sometimes we must get lost before we discover a beautiful path we didn't see before. Author John O'Donohue[17] believes that deep within each of us is an unprotected place where beauty always dwells, and we can reach it if we quiet our minds to rest in serenity. Stepping out in nature to observe just one thing can help us refocus from loss to beauty.

Standing by the ocean watching the rhythm of the waves, while adjusting our breath to become slow and deep, will go a long way toward inviting serenity. Nature has a way of coaxing us deeply inward. If we must remain indoors, we can appreciate the artistry of a pottery mug holding our favorite hot beverage, or the blooms and deep green leaves of an indoor plant. We can sit by a window and watch the wind in the trees, cloud patterns, people or wildlife activity.

Finding beauty has a lot to do with attitude, so if we are determined that there is no beauty around us, that is exactly what we will see. If we cultivate a style of mind that can reach through turbulence to an inner stillness, our own serenity will permeate our seeing, so the way we look at things changes. How we see determines what we see. When we look for beauty, we will discover it in the most unexpected places, and soon we will delight in seeing it everywhere.

Our life is enlarged when we experience beauty. We recognize the unique in the ordinary, and what was taken for granted becomes a gift. When we become calm and serene, we enter our own inner beauty which gives us a glow that no cosmetic can imitate. Beauty is the presence that waits for the expectant heart. Stepping outside of busyness and seeking beauty awakens what is concealed, and is a gift to you and everyone around you. May your heart feel the embrace of beauty wherever you find it.

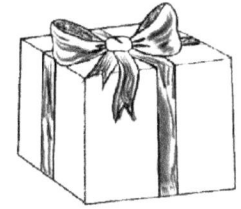

GRACE IS A GIFT WE ALL RECEIVE

Grace is a nourishing gift life gives us on a daily basis. This is the generosity of life meeting our needs abundantly, often from unexpected sources. It isn't something we work for or earn - it's given free of any requirements. Thomas Adams wrote this about grace, "Grace comes into the soul, as the morning sun into the world; first a dawning; then a light; and at last, the sun in its full and excellent brightness."[18] Once we begin recognizing grace, we will see it everywhere. Grace is both inside and all around us.

Grace is when we get an unexpected check in the mail that meets an immediate need, a visitor that comes when we're sick, holds our hand, and knows not to stay too long, a meal delivered by a neighbor when life is overwhelming us, or finding the right doctor in an emergency. Grace lives in the love between two people, especially when they are generous with forgiveness. Forgiveness is grace in action. When one stranger helps another, or we hear of a job opening from an unexpected source, that too is grace. It's the thoughtful people that show up in a crisis, or the conversation with a friend that nourishes us. Grace is there every time we seek guidance from our Higher Power.

When we live in grace, we can't help but live in gratitude as well. The stress and busyness of our everyday lives can lead to frustration when we get carried away with our to-do lists. Living in a state of grace and gratitude enhances our clarity, so we let go of what isn't serving us well and navigate stress in a healthier way. Grace builds authenticity because we understand who we really are, and when we're truly ourself it's an invitation to others to be truly themselves. This builds richer relationships and brings more peace into our life. Caroline Myss writes, "Grace is a power that comes in and transforms a moment into something better."[19]

There is so much more to life than meets the eye and grace is part of that. What can we do to invite more grace into our life? We can let go of what we can't control and surrender to whatever we call our Higher Power, which may be God, Great Spirit, Universe or even life itself. Grace is there every time we seek help. Our thoughts speak to our brain, but our inner spirit speaks to our hearts with love and guidance, so let's listen to our heart's recognition of grace.

We invite grace when we live in love, kindness and compassion. Living simply creates a sanctuary for grace in both our heart and home, and spending time in nature focuses us on the beauty of the natural world. We see grace easily when we live in truth and avoid the dishonesty that destroys trust in a relationship.

Living in the present moment enables us not to miss the small gifts of grace that are right in front of us like a sudden opening in traffic, or the person that invites us to go ahead of them in a store checkout line. Anne Lamott writes, "I do not at all understand the mystery of grace – only that it meets us where we are but does not leave us where it found us."[20] When we open our eyes to its presence, it can be seen everywhere.

Grace is what sustains us through our most difficult times. Sometimes we fight and struggle with what life is giving us, but when we give that up, we can settle into graceful living where our hearts are filled with peace and gratitude. Grace gives us hope and allows us to trust that no matter what happens, our needs will be met. Thomas Adams wrote the song "Amazing Grace" and one line from the song is this, "Through many dangers, toils and snares, I have already come; 'Tis grace has brought me safe thus far and grace will lead me home."[21] Let's be led home to the benevolent heart, generosity of spirit and unconditional love that is ours through grace. Welcome home.

INTUITION – OUR INNER GPS

The last time my husband and I purchased a car, both of us made a list of what functions were most important to us. Knowing my talent for getting lost meant an onboard GPS system was at the top of my list. That was one item we could easily agree on, so it was part of our new car. Now a voice we have named Lois, kindly tells us exactly where we are, and how to get to where we want to be. If we deviate from her instructions there is silence, and then a new route is suggested to get us back on track. If I listen to Lois, I know exactly where I am and how to get to where I need to go.

Even more exciting is the knowledge that inside each of us is an inner GPS navigator. But, for some reason it's harder to trust our inner GPS than the one we have in our car. Maybe it's because Lois's voice is very clear and distinct, and our inner guidance often comes softly. Listening and trusting take practice. It's the proverbial still small voice that we call our instinct, intuition, gut feeling, inner nudge, or sixth sense. Mark Nepo writes this about intuition, "The way we think and feel and sense our way into all we don't know is the art of intuition. It is an art of discovery. To intuit means to look upon, to instruct from within, to understand or learn by instinct. And instinct refers to a learning we are born with. So intuition is a very personal way we learn to listen to the Universe in order to discover the knowledge we are born with."[22]

 As we begin to still our minds, we can learn to listen and trust. We become adept at receiving and fine tuning the constantly transmitted signals that are there for our guidance. A friend, who practices acupuncture, told me this personal story the last time I worked with her. A mole developed on her that grew quickly, looked strange, and bled with the slightest bump. She immediately sensed something was wrong and went to her dermatologist, who blew it off as unimportant. A couple of weeks later she returned to her dermatologist asking for a biopsy. She was again blown off and refused a biopsy. At that point, my friend knew she needed a new dermatologist. Only by sticking with her inner knowing that she needed a biopsy, and pursuing a new doctor, did she get her needs met. And yes, her biopsy showed her mole was quickly turning into cancer.

My intuition has repeatedly helped me when I'm driving. I've lost track of the number of times that I have been in traffic, and suddenly known the car just ahead of me in the next lane is going to switch lanes. Without any signal, or even a head-turn from the driver, the car cut right in front of me. I had just enough time to slow down and prevent an accident only because I had an inner warning.

Intuition is creative in the way it communicates. It can be what physicians sometimes call "the educated gut." That is a visceral feeling that is a physical reaction in the center of our bodies which can't be denied. It's telling us to stop and evaluate. It can be a nudge to try something new which broadens our horizons. Or it can be a sudden realization that we are putting ourselves in danger and we need to leave the situation. It also offers a clear directive in choosing activities, clarifying when to say "yes" or "no" so we choose what is healthy or safe for us. Sometimes it is the inner knowing that we are in the right place at the right time, and we are surrounded by a synchronicity of affirming events.

But sometimes we have trouble trusting our own judgement, so trusting our inner nudges is even more difficult. Something may have felt right at the time, but later turned out to be a mistake. A person we thought we could trust was dishonest and manipulative. That not only shakes our trust in the other person, but we wonder how we could have been so mistaken, we question if we can trust ourselves again. I certainly don't have all the answers, but I wonder if what I call mistakes weren't actually important lessons that needed to happen at that point in time. Now I look back at my past with gratitude because I'm not sure I would have learned those lessons any other way. Without trust in our intuition, we live in fear, which impairs our judgement. If we take time to look at what we gained by our so called mistake, we will fear less, trust more, and live in gratitude.

Today, let's tune into the intuitive sense endowed to us by our Higher Power to help us navigate the maze of life. Let's quietly go within so we can hear the soft whispers, and feel the gentle nudges of our instincts. Let's take that leap of faith and trust our gut feeling. If we need to, we can begin small, and gradually build our inner GPS listening skills into the strong guidance system it is meant to be.

JUST GIVE IT A LITTLE HUG

After selecting some new towels, my husband and I were standing in line at a home goods retailer. Our turn to check out came, our order was rung up, and my husband inserted his credit card for payment. The long narrow card reader rejected his card three times. This had never happened before. The woman cashiering asked for his card while she described how fussy this reader was. Sometimes a speck of dust would set it off so she carefully wiped Curt's card and handed it back to him. Then she cupped one hand around the top of the card reader and said, "Sometimes we need to just give it a little hug. Now try your card again." This time the card was read and the transaction was completed.

Her phrase, "just give it a little hug" and the positive attitude that went with it, stayed with me and became the focus of our conversation driving home. Hugging people is one of my favorite things to do but hugging an inanimate object, as a way of asking for its cooperation, never occurred to me. The cashier's phrase made me wonder if that wouldn't be a good problem-solving skill to use whatever the issue might be. What if I spent more time embracing my challenges instead of complaining – would it make a difference?

My sister Paula and I are both "computer challenged". Computer logic is so far from our logic that problem solving produces high levels of stress, colorful language, and the desire to throw the computer into the nearest trash container. One day Paula, after verbally abusing her computer, reached the throwing point and called a computer technician to her house. The young man arrived and the first thing he did was talk to the machine telling it that it would feel better soon. Then he patted it, and began to softly sing to it while he worked, using only positive words. In short order her computer was running smoothly again. Paula realized her negative attitude was part of the problem. We're both working on embracing our challenges and improving our language and attitude with ever changing technology. After all; who needs more stress?

We know from years of research that physical hugs are more than just pleasurable. When we hold someone in our arms, we create a bond that leads to stress release and muscle relaxation. Hugs increase dopamine and serotonin levels so they are an instant mood booster. Since hugs elevate mood, it also helps relieve depression. Studies show that people who hug frequently have stronger immune systems than those with few hugs. Hugs can even help reduce pain because endorphins, that help block pain pathways to the brain, are released. This is why massage feels so good – it's an all over body hug!

Sometimes hugs work when words fail. Our feelings are exchanged through touch so empathy, understanding and love are received through the release of oxytocin, which is sometimes called the love hormone. Hugs tell us we are not alone. Hugs can help slow a racing heart which is what I get when I have to speak in public. I now know what to do before speaking.

Whether it's a precious person or an inanimate object, we can change the atmosphere around what is happening with a kind attitude and gentle hug. Embracing challenges instead of complaining does make a difference. Next time we're challenged let's" just give it a little hug."

KEEPING THE LIGHT BULB CONNECTED

In his book titled **Falling Upward**, Richard Rohr[23] describes a conversation he had with Desmond Tutu when they were together in Cape Town. They were talking about the need for a guiding light when Desmond Tutu said, "We are only the light bulbs, Richard, and our job is just to remain screwed in."

Staying connected – that's the secret for light bulbs and people. When we align ourselves with the high vibrations of positive energy we invite love, synchronicity, gratitude, and healthy choices into our life. We're able to honor and respect ourselves. Living in love offers the highest vibrational frequency for the best connection. Dr. David R. Hawkins writes, "Love is a state of being – it is a forgiving, nurturing and supporting way of relating to the world…..It has the capacity to lift others and accomplish great feats because of its purity of motive."[24]

The opposite of living in love is living in fear. Fear lowers our energy, promoting doubt and worry, which sabotage our ability to stay connected. This low energy attracts more low energy until we are completely disconnected, and our personal power is diminished. It's through our thoughts that we choose love or fear, so one important way to stay "screwed in" is to monitor the messages we are giving ourselves.

One of the most important ways to bring a guiding light to our lives is to trust in something greater than ourselves. When we're connected it doesn't matter if we call it the Great Spirit, Higher Self, Universe, Divine Being, God, or any other name. Alexander Graham Bell said, "What this power is I cannot say. All I know is that it exists."[25] This positive energy enhances every aspect of life and, as our path is illuminated, we see clearly and others receive the light that overflows. We can ask for guidance and help. What a relief – we don't have to do all the work.

Respecting and honoring ourselves is another way to turn on our guiding light. Let's check our choices and make sure they promote physical, mental, spiritual, and emotional good health. Let's leave past mistakes in the past so they don't sabotage the present. When something doesn't feel right let's give it the time it needs for clarity. And let's check again to make sure we are living in love, not fear.

Another powerful frequency is gratitude. Connecting to gratitude lights up our lives and becomes a beautiful circle for attracting more high energy. Gratitude turns a little into abundance, a meal into a feast, and a difficult experience into a gift. When we start looking at all the gifts there are in our lives, we start to see the gift in everything. And when we do this, no matter what is happening, our quality of life escalates, positive energy naturally flows, and our light shines.

Another positive connection is found when we choose nourishing relationships. These are full of love, gratitude, support, and respect. This honors the light in all of us so choices and concerns can be shared. The message from Richard Rohr and Desmond Tutu is to stay connected ("screwed in") and the light will take care of everything else. Keep shining!

SEEING WITH THE HEART

There is so much more to life than meets the outer eye. A deeper vision is possible when we see with the heart. Heart vision takes us below the surface and affects how we respond to what is unappealing in ourself and others. It changes our decision making, allows us to connect to our deepest self, and influences the priorities we choose. Anytime we see a situation or a person that is unpleasant to the eye, and recognize that there is more to the story then what I see, we are beginning to see with our heart's eyes.

One of our neighborhood security guards has serious facial burns that were my focus when I first saw him. Then I noticed the sparkling eyes and winning personality that made him delightful, and my attention was no longer on his burns. It was a switch from seeing him with my eyes, to seeing him with my heart. There are also scars we carry inside ourself that defy how well we may look outside. These scars are harder to see – especially when they are our own. They can only be seen with gentle heart vision. Antoine de Saint-Exupery wrote, "It is only with the heart that one can see rightly; what is essential is invisible to the eye.".[26]

None of us get through life without tough challenges. Our inner vision is a critical tool for seeing below the surface, and treating ourself and others with compassion. It takes courage to open our hearts and see with our heart's eyes. As we consciously practice, little by little our heart vision is awarded access to the power of love. The deeper we go, the more we sense the endless energy of love that transforms everything we see. It takes us to our Higher Power where we have everything we need for clear vision and guidance.

There are simple things we can do to get to that deeper place. We can step back from stimulation and spend time in solitude and silence. It's easier to see with our heart when we're calm and centered, which means not overplanning our day. Comforting words to ourself and slow deep breathing can sooth us when we're upset. This allows us to become receptive instead of reactive. We go deeper when we honor our feelings by acknowledging them, and crying when needed. Taking the risk to be vulnerable with people we trust also improves our heart vision. When we silence our inner critic, we relieve ourself from feelings of inadequacy that can block our ability to see deeper. It helps to slow down enough to find beauty throughout our day. This invites deep, rich experiences to come through our heart's eyes and into our life.

The result of heart vision can be seen in our behavior. When we see with our heart, we truly listen to each other, and if differing opinions are shared it's done without vilifying anyone. Being right is not the goal, so no judgement needs to happen. We acknowledge the nudges and messages we're receiving from our heart and act on them. Another sign is empathizing with others so we gain their perspective. Showing kindness is evident as well as daily gratitude. Compassion comes from the heart when we acknowledge we're all doing the best we can with what we have to work with.

This is about looking at the world and our experiences with different eyes. It's a process that needs patience as small shifts happen when we're ready. As we allow the process of seeing with our heart's eyes to unfold, we will see our heart vision is leading us exactly where we need to go. The world will never be the same and neither will we. When we see below the surface and discover a depth of vision only available through the heart's eyes, life can become more incredible than we ever imagined.

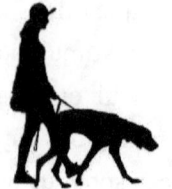

SMALL CHANGES MAKE A DIFFERENCE

In the past, January used to inspire me to make resolutions for major changes. Then I wondered why it all fizzled out by the end of February. Now I know it was because I tried to do too much at once so change wasn't sustainable. The discovery that small changes can still make a difference is helpful because those little shifts can affect our health, happiness, community, relationships and environment.

Health and happiness begin by paying attention to our thoughts. Since we choose our thoughts, it's important to remember that our thoughts affect our feelings, and feelings affect our behavior. Let's choose to stay away from negativity, fear, and the need to be right, and instead focus on the positive energy found in changing what we can, and accepting what we can't. Our bodies and minds will thank us.

We all know the importance of exercise, but not all of us can do a heavy workout in a gym. It's good to know there are benefits found in as little as twenty minutes of walking three times a week. Starting the day with a series of stretches helps us gently wake up our minds and bodies. We can walk when taking a phone call, park further away from the store, and stretch and stroll around the office once an hour. When watching a movie, we can do tasks or move around the house during commercial breaks. There's thirty-five minutes of movement opportunity in every 2-hour movie. Playing with children, walking the dog, dancing and yoga count too. Every movement counts.

Our diet is improved with every fruit and vegetable we eat, so let's try adding just one more of each a day. Setting a bowl of fruit on the kitchen counter makes it easy to reach so it's easier to avoid less healthy alternatives. A glass of water or a mug of hot lemon water first thing in the morning helps gently get our inner body systems going. Mindful eating throughout the day will keep us energized and productive. When we're out we can carry nuts or mandarin oranges to give an energy boost in between meals.

Small changes that help relationships begin by taking care of ourself first. If we do what we love to do, even if others think we should be doing something else, we will thrive. I had a university teacher who tried to discourage me from going into teaching by repeatedly saying it was a poor choice, and I would never get a job in my city. I paid no attention, followed my heart and soon had two job offers. Another helpful change is establishing an early morning and bedtime routine that begins and ends our day in a nurturing way. Computers, phones and news are not helpful at either time. A gratitude journal is a great way to end the day on a positive note, especially if the day's been hard. Writing just one thing down can make a difference in what we focus on as we go to sleep.

The biggest gift we can give to others is to listen well. That means putting our smartphone on "airplane" mode, giving the speaker eye contact, and weighing our attitude and words before we respond. We can reach out to one person every day with a call or text, or write a thank you note to someone who has impacted our life.

Our communities are affected by small changes such as going for a walk with a trash bag to pick up litter, which may inspire others to do the same. Just saying "Hi" to neighbors creates a friendly atmosphere, and making soup for someone who is ill, builds caring neighborhoods. In our neighborhood we keep in touch with each other so we know if someone needs help. Donating to a charity doesn't need to involve a large amount of money. Our local food banks can make a small donation go a long way.

Our environment is helped by going vegetarian for a day or more to relieve the demand for meat. We can use leftover drinking water to water plants or purchase a water saving shower head. Keeping reusable grocery bags in our car means we're more likely to use them. We can slowly replace our regular light bulbs with LED bulbs which last longer and use less energy. If every American household replaced just one bulb a year, the pollution reduction would be equivalent to removing over 2 million cars from the road every year.

Minor changes are easy and can affect every area of our personal life, community and environment. Try one and see what happens. Small changes really do make a difference.

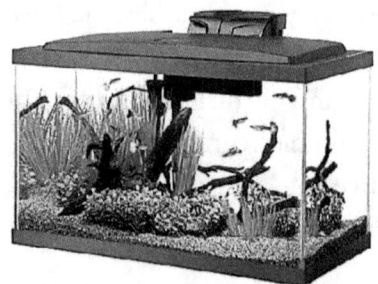

SOOTHING SIMPLICITY

Living simply is a refreshing perspective on life that can transform us from living with the tyranny of the urgent, to living with mindful decisions and peaceful attitudes. Choosing simplicity means letting go of whatever does not add value to our life, so we can focus on what we truly love. It's trading superficiality, noise and excess, for contentment, gratitude and meaning.

Soothing simplicity isn't hard to achieve because it begins with small steps. Here are a few suggestions. Henry Ward Beecher reminds us that, "The first hour of the morning is the rudder of the day."[27] How we start our day sets the tone for the rest of the day, so let's give ourselves some precious morning quiet time to focus on what's most important. When we clarify our priorities, we can let go of everything else. This creates the best possible frame of mind. I like to start my day with a prayer of gratitude, so I continue to be grateful throughout the day. A simple evening routine helps us unwind when we choose activities that are relaxing and calming. This prepares us for a peaceful night's sleep.

Our environment is simplified by getting rid of clutter, so what we have is organized and easily accessed. Having a budget clarifies where the money is going and what needs changing. Multitasking does not fit into simplicity so that needs to go. It also helps to remove the "just in case" concept from our life – all those things we keep in case we might need them. We can avoid becoming a hoarder by buying only what we need at the time we need it.

Prioritizing self-care is an important part of soothing simplicity. We take care of ourself when we say no to requests that are not right for us. Paying attention to our health and fitness means we can cut down on those props we use to relieve stress like sugar, snack foods, or alcohol. Eliminating toxic people opens up space in our life. Decluttering our relationships allows us to focus our time on nurturing relationships that feature mutual love, respect and support.

Simplicity calls for down time which means time away from our phones and computers. It means getting comfortable with doing nothing. I like to watch cloud shapes change, the wind in the trees, or listen to bird songs outside our front door. My husband has an aquarium screen saver that he watches to reel himself in whenever he's lost himself in busyness. When we practice mindfulness, we stay in the moment and center ourself so we stay grounded in what means most to us. Getting out in nature always helps restore calm and balance.

There are benefits to living simply and they begin with reduced stress. Letting go of everything we don't need is freeing, so we experience more peace of mind. Simplifying gives us quality over quantity and clarity over chaos. It helps us save money so we have more financial freedom. We are freed from being possessed by our possessions and all the time it takes to maintain them. Simplicity frees us from comparing ourself to others. We are more productive because we are less distracted. Simplifying allows us to be content with less because we have defined how much is enough. We're able to live more deliberately because we are focused on the present moment. And we're able to do more of what we love so life satisfaction increases.

John Burroughs writes, "To find the universal elements enough; to find the air and water exhilarating; to be refreshed by a morning walk or an evening saunter....to be thrilled by the stars at night; to be elated over a bird's nest or a wildflower in spring – these are some of the rewards of the simple life."[28]

The process of simplifying is a journey. What worked before may need to be reconsidered as our environment, health, or needs change. Just know that whatever steps we take to simplify, we'll be rewarded with increased calmness and a richer life experience. Simplicity helps us realize we already have everything we need for contentment.

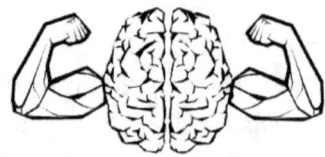

STAYING MENTALLY STRONG IN TOUGH TIMES

Whatever form it takes, we all have times when life becomes difficult. Today there are many stressors so mental health is more important than ever. Staying mentally strong gives us what we need to navigate challenges successfully. Just like steadily building physical strength over time results in strong muscles, steadily building mental strength results in navigating our tough times with clarity and resiliency.

Amy Morin, psychotherapist, mental strength coach, and author of the book "*13 Things Mentally Strong People Don't Do*,"[29] discovered in her research what strategies mentally strong people use when life pushes them the hardest. Right now, let's give our mental health some attention, and look at some of her healthy coping skills that can help us manage our thoughts, feelings, and behaviors.

Acknowledging our inner strength is essential because choosing to believe that we'll never get through a situation, insures our inability to cope. Mentally strong people remind themselves that they're capable, even if answers aren't yet clear. Self-talk is kind instead of judgmental. Our inner strength is enhanced by a strong spiritual practice that focuses on the kind of love and compassion that celebrates the humanity of everyone. Meditation is used for present moment awareness, a calm mind, and stability.

Accepting reality keeps us mentally strong because we are acknowledging what is happening – whether we like it or not. What is, is! This reality helps us see where we have control so we can decide how to respond. Our resources are focused on what is needed to keep us healthy and safe. For all those things that are out of our control, the only thing we can change is our attitude about them.

We strengthen mentally when we release ourselves from rigid thinking that says there's only one solution to a problem, or a situation must turn out a certain way. When we remain flexible, we're able to adapt to new challenges, and see more options. We don't sweat the small stuff so petty annoyances won't ruin our day. The focus is on what matters most, so strength is saved for the important issues that yield meaningful results.

Mentally strong people admit their mistakes, but don't hyper focus on their failures. Instead, they focus in on what can be done differently. Maya Angelou writes, "You may encounter many defeats, but you must not be defeated. In fact, it may be necessary to encounter the defeats, so you can know who you are, what you can rise from, how you can still come out of it."[30]

Trying something new can feel daunting, but mentally strong people know that changing course may be the only way to move ahead. Avoiding anything new keeps us stuck in a difficult place. Small incremental successes can build the confidence and comfort needed for major changes. That's building mental muscle before a crisis. Taking action is also part of creating mental strength. If a problem can't be solved, (like a serious illness or passing of a loved one) choices are made to cope with the distress in healthy ways.

Mentally healthy people practice gratitude, even when life is difficult. This is not denying pain or minimizing hardship, but along with that there is also finding things to be grateful for in the middle of a trying time. Sometimes gratitude comes from reflecting on what we've learned in our darkest hour. Some of our greatest insights are gained from the toughest challenges, and the value of these insights will stay with us the rest of our life.

Building mental muscle also involves not taking everything personally. Social media gives us the opportunity to be goaded into arguments with complete strangers. Instagram photos can make everyone else look like their doing great while we're struggling. Mentally strong people focus on their goals and avoid the negative distractions that can be part of Twitter and Snapchat. Obstacles or setbacks are not taken personally because we recognize our own worth is not attached to whatever needs changing.

Let's keep building our mental strength so we have what we need when we're tested. As always, we learn through challenges so we're learning on the job. Paying attention to our mental strength helps us emerge from a struggle with new perspective, strength and confidence. That makes it worth all the hard work.

THE RHYTHM OF LIFE – CAN YOU FEEL IT?

"If you study the rhythm of life on this planet, you will find that everything moves in perfect symphony with everything else – by grand divine design. The earth has the ability to heal and regenerate itself, just as our oceans have the ability to replenish themselves by turning over their debris with the waves that wash it ashore. This perfect orchestration of the cycle of life is one of the Creator's greatest and most beautiful miracles."[31] (Suzy Kassem) Everything about us including our mind, body, and spirit, is a part of the rhythm of life's cycles. And all nature, such as plants, trees, oceans, animals, and birds, have their steady rhythmic cycle.

The rhythm of life that nature obeys is seen in the ebb and flow of tides that follow a monthly pattern tied to the sun and moon's gravitational pull. Recently I read that air temperature determines the rhythmic timing of the cricket's chirp. We have all watched large groups of birds obeying their inner rhythm that tells them where, and when, to fly for needed climate and food. Even sun flowers have a circadian rhythm that guides them to begin the day facing east and finish the day facing west. This points towards the rhythm of sunrise and sunset.

The authors like Mark Nepo, in their writings suggest that every form of life goes through the process of emerging, coming together, creating new life, falling apart, dying and reemerging in a new way. Just as nature has its seasons throughout the year, our individual experiences form their own similar seasons creating our personal ebb and flow. The rhythm of life, death, and rebirth, is universal.

How do we feel and listen to the rhythm of our lives? Rob Bell offers a good place to start, "You just took a breath. You're about to take another. Inhale, then exhale, then another inhale. In and out. There's a rhythm in your breathing."[32] Add to that the rhythm of our heart beat, and the comforting daily cycles of sleep and awake, rest and play, solitude and social time, and eating at regular intervals.

The more sensitive we are to our personal rhythms, the more effective we can be in determining what we need. When our daily lives with their regular routines are interrupted by change, we are given the opportunity to experience a new rhythm, and learn that we are stronger and more durable than we may think. Whether static or changing, the rhythm of life is the powerful beat under all that happens. Enjoy its cadence, honor its presence, and feel the joy of your individual rhythm. Take this advice from Mehmet Murat who writes, "Don't let anybody ruin your inner joy or interfere in your marvelous rhythm!"[33]

If we embrace the ebb and flow of our days, we are honoring the tempo of our lives. This makes us happier, more productive, less stressed, and grateful for what each day brings. We know when darkness comes light will follow, as joy will follow sorrow. Let's feel the rhythm of our life, and celebrate how far we've come - how healing it is to connect with others in this personal way. May we feel the perfect harmony of our life's rhythm and know that, whenever changes occur, there will always be beauty in the beat of your sacred dance.

YOU ARE AN ARTIST

Whenever I watch my husband paint, I marvel at his ability to look at something and reproduce it on canvas. That is a talent I do not have! During my teaching years there were times when I wanted to illustrate something on the white board, so I would draw stick figures. The students and I would laugh at my silly drawings, but I was keeping their attention which was the goal. However, drawing and painting are only one form of art. Slowly, through time and experience, I realized the opportunities to be an artist were many and varied. Let's look at a broadened perspective.

We are all artists simply by the fact that we are here on the planet. Our life is a work in progress which means we are offered a fresh canvas every morning. We can rewrite, redo, change color, edit, or start all over again each day. Sarah Ban Breathnach writes, "Art evolves. So does life. Art is never stagnant. Neither is life. The beautiful, authentic life you are creating for yourself and those you love is your art. It's the highest art."[34]

An artist is someone who is carefully listening to their inner inspiration, which comes from the creative energy of the Universe. Every daily choice becomes part of the tug between taking a risk, or playing it safe. What would we like to do different today than we did yesterday? Is there something new we'd like to try? Sarah Ban Breathnach offers this thought, "Each time you experience the new, you become receptive to inspiration. Each time you try something different, you let the Universe know you are listening. Trust your instincts. Believe your yearnings are blessings. Respect your creative urges."[35]

Well done art takes thought and preparation. Our presence, our voice, our truth is needed in whatever form we can give. Stories of survival and triumph take on new beauty because of the courage and bravery on our daily canvas. Those of us with serious physical challenges understand the bright color, rough texture, and continually evolving shape of our lives. We create each day with patient longing and flexible emotion, solid hope and silent prayer, positive (or negative) attitude and inner discernment. We create with healing tears, red scars, and sore raw skin. We create with the constant change illness or injury brings, so what worked one day may not work the next. Leslie Odom Jr. writes, "One of the things I know for sure is: the issues of your life effect your work and the issues found in your work are showing up somewhere else in your life. This is a spiritual walk as well. Ask the questions. Go in search of the answers."[36] Creative living is a daily artistic miracle.

Often artists are unsung, but that does not diminish their art. Beauty does not depend on accolades. Each of us is working on what is uniquely ours to produce, and that means we are participating in the art of living. Meg Black writes, "I realized that it did not matter how old I was or how much money I needed or what people might think of my new efforts, I was in fact an artist, made by a greater power (in my case God) to be creative. What I am saying is that there is a spiritual energy available to all of us. It is in our DNA and all we have to do is activate it and use it."[37] Since we only have one life, let's make our living on this planet a masterpiece of endeavor. It doesn't matter if we make mistakes, that's all part of art. It's the doing that grows our souls.

I'd like to end with this quote from Tsh Oxenreider. "As you start this week, may you find a nugget of courage to do the hard thing your heart is aching to do. May you find enough freedom to do something brave and risky, something that taps that gift you were given but haven't yet fully and outwardly exercised. We are all artists in some way, whether our media is watercolor, keyboard, food, camera, numbers, or diaper. What is the main thing keeping you from doing your art – is it time, money, courage, or encouragement? Do you have a voice this week telling you that your work isn't important? May you combat lies with truth this week and may you dare to be you, in small ways and big. May you look in the mirror and in the words of your journal and love who you truly are. And may you find enough courage to acknowledge your artistry, and to recognize the ways your life teems with canvases."[38]

Chapter 3 - Insights Into Ourselves

BALANCE – WHERE ARE YOU?

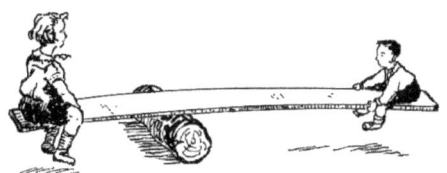

This morning my body was complaining loudly enough that I knew I needed to stay home today. After cancelling participation in an activity I normally enjoy, I knew I needed to revisit activities for the weekend, too. While my stomach rolled and my body hurt, my intuition was waving a red flag. This was familiar territory and, having a history of learning the hard way, I decided to restore balance now.

If the goal is balance, then we need to take into account all of our needs. We need balance between work and play, thoughts and feelings, our professional and personal life, giving and receiving, the physical and spiritual realm, family and personal needs. There is a still, small voice of spiritual guidance that alerts us when change is required. However, we need to be listening to this guidance. The more we listen the easier it is to pick up on the gentle inner nudging's that offer guidance, to the right time and place, through a flow of synchronicity. Katherine Butler Hathaway shares this thought on intuition: "It is only by following your deepest instinct that you can lead a rich life and if you let your fear of consequence prevent you from following your deepest instinct then your life will be safe, expedient, and thin."[1]

Intuition offers balance and balance promotes harmony. Here is a musical analogy. Think of a Chopin piano concerto played by a novice musician compared to a virtuoso. Both are playing the same notes, but one of them has had a lifetime of practice and knows exactly where to pause in order to create meaning and passion to the piece. If we look at our lives as a concerto, then we know individual notes must be learned, played, and practiced to produce the balanced harmony of our passion. Even more important is knowing when to pause! There is an inner cadence of contentment when we have struck just the right balance between our family and community responsibilities, and our inner needs for spiritual growth and personal expression.

Sarah Ban Breathnach offers this insight, "Usually, when the distractions of daily life deplete our energy, the first thing we eliminate is the thing we need the most: quiet, reflective time. Time to dream, time to think, time to contemplate what's working and what's not, so we can make changes for the better."[2] Often it is the pause in music that gives it meaning and beauty, and it is the pauses in life that guide us into the harmony of daily balance.

Today I'm slowing down to reevaluate what I need to change. I'm wanting to avoid a noisy cacophony of demands, in favor of a symphony from my soul – that is where balance resides. Finding our balance everyday keeps us in harmony with our priorities, promoting health and contentment. May your day hold the notes and pauses of balance.

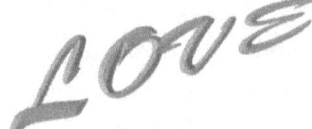

CLAIMING OUR PERSONAL POWER

When the unexpected happens it's easy to become overwhelmed and forget the power we have through the choices we make. Real power isn't about dominance over someone else, it's about clarifying what is most important to us and making decisions based on that. It's about the energy and creativity that happen when self-understanding grows and insights deepen because we're connected to the most powerful energy there is – love. Love makes what we do, and who we are, align. Mari Perron tells us love is all there is.[3]

We're not in control of everything that happens to us, but we are in control of how we respond. Do we want to lash out in fear, or respond with the powerful thoughts, words and actions from love's energy? Alice Walker wrote, "The most common way people give away their power is by thinking they don't have any."[4]. Feeling powerless doesn't mean we are powerless – we always have a choice.

Here are some ways we give our power away. When we believe old messages from others about not being lovable, good enough, able to solve our problems, or worthy of success, we lose power. Making decisions based on what other people will think diminishes us. Ignoring our intuition, which is our strong, loving inner guidance, works against us.

Continually putting other people's needs first, minimizing our gifts and strengths, not speaking up when something is wrong, or waiting for someone to give us permission to do what we really want to do is ignoring our power to choose differently. We also lose when we give in to guilt trips, neglect to set boundaries, hold grudges and complain. Anytime we let someone else determine the kind of day we're having we've lost our personal power.

Reclaiming our personal power is all about recognizing we have a choice. Since love is the most powerful energy there is, we can choose to live in love instead of fear, which will change our whole outlook on life. Loving ourself means we use our power to set healthy boundaries so we do what best supports us. This is especially needed when we're dealing with a serious illness or family crisis. We can set limits for visitors, fire the doctor that is unhelpful or the counselor that's unempathetic (I've done all of those). Every medical treatment is our choice, and sometimes we chose not to have treatment.

When we claim our personal power, we eliminate toxic people from our life and never tolerate abuse. Giving ourself permission to follow our heart is practicing the power to create our own life. Reclaiming happens when we remove our self-worth from the opinion of others. We can take responsibility for our emotions and let others be responsible for theirs. When a hurt happens, we can choose to forgive and move forward.

Releasing negative patterns of behavior, valuing our opinion of ourself, and living according to our guiding principles will help us live into our personal power. It happens when we clearly ask for what we need. We can choose to focus on our own gifts and talents and let go of the need to be right.

Other people's negative behavior does not need to disempower us. Our personal power increases when we understand that what is happening is a reflection of them and their emotional state, not us. We keep our power when we avoid rehashing unhelpful interactions. This is the energy of love at work.

Choices make us the driver instead of the passenger. The reality of our situation may not change, but we will change. As we practice empowering ourself, we will feel better about ourself and our choices. Feeling better is contagious so the people around us will be more empowered, too. Reclaiming our personal power is a win/win for all of us.

CREATING INNER PEACE

General Manager
The Universe

We often hear remarks about the importance of peace on the world stage, especially as it relates to war. We are taught that conflicts and battles over differences need to be fought and won. But what if we adjusted our thinking to focus on how to welcome peace, by understanding and dismantling what we are individually battling. The place to start is also the most difficult place to be, because it means taking an intimate look at ourselves, and being honest about our personal conflicts. The message here isn't about global peace, it's about the power of personal peace, which is the only way global peace will ever happen. Much can be said on this topic, and the following ideas are not comprehensive, but are suggested as a helpful reminder for creating inner peace.

As cancer survivors, we know the demanding challenge of making peace with our diseased bodies. The surgeries and drugs for our treatments all have side effects, and change the look and feel of our bodies. Some changes are temporary like hair loss, and raw skin, and some are permanent like scars, and parts of our bodies we no longer have. Recently a medical test suggested I had colon cancer. Further testing showed it was a false positive, but for three weeks I lived with the possibility of a second round of cancer. Once I made peace with possibility, there was no fear, tension, or anxiety because I knew that whatever happened, my peaceful foundation would carry me through. I would be fine no matter what my body was doing.

We need to make peace with every change, because therein lies the richness of discovering the tranquil beauty of our inner self. Sometimes we have a hard time recognizing this when we're in turmoil. It helps to face whatever form change has taken, acknowledge what we can't control, accept the feelings that emerge, and give ourselves permission to be imperfect. Serenity will follow.

Another challenge is making peace with our aging bodies. This is another place to give ourselves permission to be imperfect. Over time all the signs are there; rising cholesterol, shrinking height, undisguised bulges, elusive sleep, and more doctor recommended vitamins. My personal favorite is what I call map legs (I inherited them from my mother) that feature red and blue highways all over my legs. The highways get more crowded each year. Make peace with it, Sylvia, make peace. The aging process isn't going to stop, but if we can become at ease with it and befriend ourselves, we are moving into peace.

One of the gifts of aging is the serenity that comes when we become more of who we really are inside. We realize the priority and preciousness of peace, and can consciously choose what nurtures our minds, renews our bodies, and feeds our soul. One of the rewards of doing this is avoiding the "activity treadmill" that keeps us going faster and faster, until we go "crazy". We do not need to do more and run faster. Larry Eisenberg writes, "For peace of mind, we need to resign as **general manager of the universe.**"[5]

Then there is making peace with conflict. Often our first reaction to conflict is anxiety, not peace. If we convince ourselves that the importance of an issue is seen in the amount of time spent worrying, we will actually give power to the problem. Power to the solution is found in calmness and peace. Bringing forgiveness to the conflict invites a divine generosity that frees us from anger and bitterness. Anxiety is a choice and so is peace. It is possible to be peaceful even in the middle of chaos and unresolved problems. If we move our focus from how hard life is, to doing what we know is right for us right now, peace of mind will follow.

Here are some ways we can nurture inner peace. Let's walk in nature until our minds are quiet. Let's watch a sunset or sunrise over the ocean or lake or river until we feel soothed. Let's meditate and pray until we are calm. Let's spend time with a dear friend and feel loved. Let's be still until our perspective is balanced and our values are clear, so we behave with integrity. And let's forgive ourselves and others on a daily basis.

Another exciting element about creating inner peace is that when we take inner peace into our daily life, it begins to spread around us. As we nurture our own peace, we begin to radiate serenity that touches others, and peace becomes contagious. This is truly powerful! So, let's check in with ourselves — how do we know we're on the right track?

Peace Pilgrim writes this, "There is a criterion by which you can judge whether the thoughts you are thinking and the things you are doing are right for you. The criterion is: Have they brought you inner peace? If they have not, there is something wrong with them - - so keep seeking! If what you do has brought you inner peace, stay with what you believe is right."[6] Today, let's create more inner peace for our own selves and those around us.

DOING MORE OF WHAT TRULY MATTERS

We live in a culture where more is honored - more work, more status, more money, and more things. The message of limitlessness may sound freeing, but it can be just the opposite. Nicole Leatherman describes it as, "shackles with a chaser of stress."[7]

There is a different way of being in the world that is both simple and profound. It offers the opportunity for more peace, more clarity, more love of self and others, and more life satisfaction. This is the transformation that can happen when we intentionally give our precious time to more of what truly matters, by doing less of what is unimportant. A daily check of our priorities is helpful. We need to pay attention because our lives are full of change, so, as challenges present themselves, what truly matters can change.

Marc Lesser describes it this way, "You may, in fact, be no less engaged, but you will be less scattered and distracted, and you may accomplish more of what matters to you, more of what aligns with your deepest purpose and intention, more of what brings you satisfaction and connection with others, more of what you believe really needs to get done."[8] When we align our actions with our values, we become peaceful because our choices have been thoughtfully made. This leads to enjoying life more and stressing less.

Here are a few suggestions for zeroing in on doing more of what truly matters. Let's begin by reminding ourself that we're the only one keeping score, so we need to eliminate our habit of being self-critical. When we criticize ourself our stress response is triggered which, if it becomes a habit, can lead to inflammation and illness. We are not in competition with anyone, including ourself. Instead of focusing on the times we've messed up, let's focus on what we've done well, knowing we're capable of doing more things well.

When we're clear on our nonnegotiables, we intentionally promote what we value most. Letting go of everything that distracts us from focusing on our top priorities will naturally lead us to doing less of what isn't important. Keeping the big picture in mind will help us avoid getting caught in minutia which can eat up hours, disturb our peace, and distract us from our main focus of the day. Our phones are especially good at this. By identifying and reducing unnecessary activities, we can let the small stuff go. This is especially true if we're dealing with a crisis in our health, finances, or relationships, and need to focus all our resources on problem solving.

If we're paying attention to what's most important, we bring greater awareness to every activity, conversation, and interaction with others, making our connections more meaningful. This means choosing to single task so we are completely present, and in between tasks we can give ourself a deep breathing break, meditation time, or a restorative nap. Doing absolutely nothing is also good for renewal. Giving ourself a break increases our emotional health, promotes serenity and boosts creativity. This is how we recharge for what really matters.

We need to say "no" strategically, even to good ideas. Doing what is right for us means we'll be selective, so our focus stays on what is essential. Choosing to do less improves the quality of our endeavors. Quantity is not the goal.

Let's relieve ourself from perfection. Perfection produces stress, and diminishes life satisfaction by sucking the joy out of our day. Its high demands can keep us from loving ourself and others. And, it eats time that could be used to enjoy doing something well that's important. For many things good is good enough. Not everything needs to be great, so let's save our best efforts for what truly matters.

Forcing ourself to do what we can't fully embrace, because it isn't top priority, can leave us feeling like we've been drained by an energy vampire. When we reduce the unnecessary, we practice clarity. We accomplish more of what truly matters when we give ourself fully to the values and goals that renew us. Let's do more of what truly matters together.

EXPERIENCING EVERYDAY AWE

Even if we didn't name it at the time, we have all experienced awe. It's that feeling of being amazed, inspired, or transported by what we're experiencing. Because the experience is incredible, we can expand our vision of what is possible, and who we are in relationship to it. Awe on a big scale happened for me when I rode an elephant through the jungles of Thailand. It also happened when I stood in the Sistine Chapel in Rome, and personally experienced that magnificent art work. However, awe is also available nearer to home in everyday life.

In his book **Awestruck**, Psychologist Jonah Paquette reveals scientific studies that show experiencing awe improves relationships, decreases stress, and actually makes us happier by improving our wellbeing. He writes, "Awe blurs the line between the self and the world around us, diminishes the ego, and links us to the greater forces that surround us in the world and the larger universe."[9] So, awe brings us closer together by blurring our separateness, and enhancing our oneness. This is about more than feeling good.

Wherever our awe comes from, Paquette points to a number of benefits. Experiencing awe will reduce stress which can last a number of weeks. The evidence of a link between being outdoors, experiencing awe, and lowering stress levels, is now so strong that some doctors are actually prescribing time at a park, beach, or any green space. If illness eliminates being active, a carefully nurtured indoor plant can produce awe.

Awe experiences can increase our generosity and kindness. When we have an inspiring experience, we lose our sense of entitlement, which enhances ethical decision-making. Awe makes us feel more connected, so we're willing to help people in need and act for the greater good. Paquette writes, "By enabling us to feel connected to each other, form alliances, act generously, and explore new possibilities, it stands to reason that the story of humans would not be possible without awe."[10] We can preserve what lifts us up by taking time to journal our awesome experiences, keeping them available for further enjoyment.

Awe impacts our mood and makes us more satisfied with life. The more awe we experience, the better we feel. This means finding awe in everyday life has benefits worth pursuing. Here are a few suggestions from Paquette for enjoying every day awe. Anytime we feel ourself amazed by something, we can enhance the experience by lingering with it as long as possible. When we loose ourself in music we can choose to stay there a while, or if we experience art that takes us out of ourself, we can spend time with it instead of hurrying on to the next activity. A meaningful photo can transport us into an inspired state. Watching a colorful sunrise or sunset can fill us with awe. When we slow down, we create a space for awe to emerge.

The beauty of people working together can also create awe. Recently we took a simple flight from Sanford, Florida to Appleton, Wisconsin. My husband, the aviation expert, told me that it took about 120 professionals working together perfectly, to get our plane full of people safely between those two destinations. That's awesome.

I have an African Violet that has developed two new baby plants. I'm inspired by every new leaf, and by the fact that the mother plant is now growing its new leaves moving the mature leaves away from the new plants, so they get more nurturing light. I'm amazed by the way this plant is taking care of the new life it started.

We invite awe when we appreciate our senses. Let's take time to fully listen to the bird song, the wind in the trees, the laughter of children having fun. We can pause to fully appreciate the scent of food cooking on the stove, and savor the taste of our meals by eating slowly enough to identify all the different flavors and textures mingling together. Walking outdoors we may become inspired by natures colorful palette, or we can choose to spend time with an indoor plant that's blooming.

Starting our day with the intention of being awed by our surroundings will enhance our focus, improve mental and physical health, aid our relationships, and make us kinder, more generous people. That's an impressive list of advantages. Since it can be found in our homes, front porches, and back yards, as well as beyond, let's take time to experience this. Everyday awe awaits.

FINDING OUR INNER ZEN

According to the Dalai Lama, "The inner peace of an alert and calm mind is the source of real happiness and good health."[11] This is one way to define our inner Zen. Our lives are full of voices from news reporters and social media, emphasizing discord and chaos. Add to that an infestation of ants in the kitchen, the car breaking down again, or the diagnosis of a serious illness, and it's easy to lose our mindfulness and peaceful inner Zen. Stressful forces will always be there, but we can make our way back to the peaceful possibility that resides in every moment.

At the first sign of stress, one of the most helpful things we can do for ourselves is to take a deep, slow breath. Several deep, slow breaths are even better because deep inhaling brings in positive energy, and exhaling discharges negativity. The effect is enhanced again if we use the mental image of sending light to our fearful and painful places. We don't need to try to calm the storm; all we need to calm is ourselves. Keeping things in perspective will help us focus on what is and not imagine the worst-case scenario. Avoiding "what if" and staying with "what is" is one doorway to finding our peaceful inner Zen.

We also find our inner Zen when we do what nourishes us on a deeper level. Our nervous system is calmed when we do yoga, meditate, have a massage, or take a bath with a candle or two and soft music. A relaxed body gains clarity and perspective. Exchanging an overcrowded calendar for time gardening, reading, or conversation with a positive friend, encourages feelings of serenity.

We won't find our inner peace with pessimistic people so we need to shift our self toward positive relationships. Our relationships are a source of support and guidance, so let's nurture every loving bond we have, and leave behind the negative influences of fear filled people who push our worry buttons. As Eckhart Tolle says, "Worry pretends to be necessary but serves no useful purpose."[12] Healthy boundaries protect our energy and reduces stress which helps create inner tranquility.

Inner Zen becomes available when we give up trying to manage the world. No matter how much we would like it to be different, there are many parts of life that are out of our control. When we learn to let things go, and take life as it comes, we increase our happiness and contentment.

Mindfulness is part of finding our inner Zen and keeps us in the moment. This helps both physical and mental health. When we handle only what is happening right now (without introducing past or future) we lower our blood pressure, calm our hormones, improve gastrointestinal issues, and sleep better.

We find the tranquility of Zen when we do what we need to do without procrastinating. If there is something that needs doing, and we continually put it off, it works in the back of our mind constantly interrupting our sense of peace. Keeping our living space clean and organized is a powerful tool for serenity. It's impossible to be inwardly relaxed when we're tripping over clutter, and can't find what we need because nothing is put away. This is something that is in our control. Getting rid of messes and clutter enhances our inner Zen.

Another element in our control is our thoughts. Our thoughts dictate what we will do with our day, how we feel, and how we react to situations and people. Our thoughts create our reality, so, if we decide everything's going to be awful it will be, but if we decide life will improve, it will improve, even if our circumstances don't. Let's exchange any state of worry or distress for inner peace, and a calm mind. Finding our inner serenity is just a thought away. When we connect with our inner Zen, we can join Mary Oliver when she says, "Sometimes I need only to stand wherever I am to be blessed."[13] Your peaceful inner Zen awaits!

FINDING OUR WAY

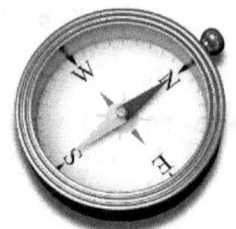

Elizabeth Kubler-Ross writes, "The most beautiful people we have known are those who have known defeat, known suffering, known struggle, known loss, and have found their way out of the depths. These persons have an appreciation, sensitivity, and an understanding of life that fills them with compassion, gentleness, and a deep loving concern. Beautiful people do not just happen."[14] If we think of life as a journey, then we know that the path isn't always clear. Today both events and people impact our lives.

Add to that finding our way through ongoing health challenges, family stress, job uncertainty, and inflation, and we may feel we're somewhere in the depths that Kubler-Ross mentions. This is an easy place to get stuck. We can get into obsessive thought patterns and lose sleep over what the future may hold. Since the future has always been unpredictable, we help ourselves when we stop overanalyzing and remember that the only place we can find our way is in the present moment.

This moment is our chance to courageously go out and create our own customized path. We grow as we bump up against limits, make mistakes, and take unexpected turns. It's then that we discover that the wrong turn was the only way we could have found the right path. Eckhart Tolle writes, "Any action is better than no action, especially if you have been stuck in an unhappy situation for a long time. If it is a mistake, at least you have learned something, in which case it's no longer a mistake. If you remain stuck you learn nothing."[15]

We find our way when we start with simple small steps; one healthy addition to our diet, one attitude change, one exercise for our body, one act of forgiveness, one action for unity, one project finished. Over time these small steps create a strong path that we could never have imagined before beginning the process. Every time we boldly take a step we clarify what the right path is for us. Our path is the sum of all those simple small steps that lead to everything we dream and do.

We find our way when we are aware of the influences around us. Since we don't live in complete isolation, we need to be sensitive to how constant "news watching" affects us, what kind of people we spend time communicating with, what our relationship is to alcohol or drugs, and what amount of time we give to meditation and spiritual practices. These are all relevant influences that can have an effect on our ability to find our way. When our next step provides us with an opportunity, we need to determine if this is a good fit, a step in the right direction.

We find our way when we believe in ourselves. This may mean saying "no" to what other people think we should be doing with our life. This is our path, not theirs, so let's avoid the seeds of self-doubt. Part of believing in ourselves is listening to our inner guidance that knows what we need most. The more we do this the better we become at hearing its voice. To do this we must be quiet. It's hard to hear one voice in a noisy crowd, so we need to step away from busyness to listen.

We find our way when we know what fulfills us. This is learned through personal growth and development until our priorities are clear, and we are able to live fully expressing our gifts. If something feels meaningful, joyful, and inspired, it is a "path finder clue" to be followed. The question I most often ask is, "Is this worth my precious life energy?" If it is, it's worth pursuing. When we wake up each morning with a spirit of gratitude for another day, we are living in fulfillment no matter what tasks the day may hold. We each have our own timeline for finding our way to what fulfills us, so we need to be patient with each other. Rumi sums it up best, "If light is in your heart you will find your way home."[16]

We all go through major events. As Kubler Ross wrote above, let's take comfort knowing that we're finding our way out of this difficult time and becoming more deeply loving, compassionate, and gentle because of it. We're finding our way into more appreciation, sensitivity and understanding. We're finding new inner strength and peace. We're leaving fear for love, and division for unity. Take solace in knowing we are finding our way.

FLAWED BEAUTY

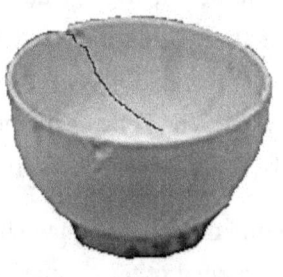

In Japan there is an art form called Wabi-sabi that celebrates imperfect beauty. Pottery bowls are intentionally created to be rustic and simple looking, with shapes that are not quite symmetrical, and textures that look unrefined. Often there is a chip in the bottom of the bowl. This is not poor workmanship, but a piece masterfully done with thoughtful planning and careful glazing. It's a celebration of imperfection – an honoring of the flaw's beauty. I'd like to suggest that we are like the Chinese bowls with our beauty intentionally planned to include all our flaws.

Embracing our humanness means accepting our flaws and finding within them a beauty beyond our culture's description of attractive. The simple truth is that no one is perfect, and striving for perfection is like a dog chasing its tail. Catching it is impossible. It's our individual uniqueness, including our flaws, that's important to true beauty, not perfection. As Brené Brown says, "Imperfections are not inadequacies; they are reminders we are all in this together."[17]

It's the parts of ourself that we don't like that have the most to teach us. Our imperfections help us make needed change. They show us how to appreciate, accept, and forgive ourself and others, creating the beauty of transformation. It's the flaw that takes us to places we would not otherwise go, leading us to deeper self-knowledge and meaningful growth. When we look at our imperfections with compassion, we become more generous in our view of others. Compassion frees us to make healthier choices, which makes the flaw a beautiful stepping stone toward fully embracing ourselves.

Sometimes we carry emotional scars that feel like flaws. It only takes one traumatic event to change our life and make it difficult to trust or love again. Often, we want to hide these scars, but with patience and an understanding counselor we can be healed. This gives meaning to the scar.

During the Olympic games Simone Biles, the most decorated gymnast in history, chose to withdraw from final performances because of mental health concerns. What may have looked like a flaw was actually a courageous stand for the needs of athletes performing under tremendous pressure. She is helping to change how athletes are being treated by the Olympic committee, the press, and social media. Her vulnerability made a strong statement as she said we are not "just athletes, we're people at the end of the day."[18] This represents the beauty of being true to oneself in a challenging situation. It's the chip in the bottom of the bowl that makes us all human.

I suspect we all have a list of what we would consider our physical flaws. My mother-in-law has decided that in her next life she is going to have smaller feet, a smaller nose, and smaller ears. I have two long surgical scars that I hoped would be fine white lines by now. They continue to be red and anything but fine. Then I remind myself that those scars represent surgery that saved my life, and the fact that I have life written in scars all over my body needs to be celebrated. They are the physical evidence that support my continued enjoyment of life. There is beauty in that.

Whatever features we have that are not celebrated by society are not a flaw – they're our own personal statement of surviving. Let's not compare ourself to others, particularly those of us who have had multiple surgeries, endured difficult treatments, or lost body parts. Instead let's embrace the flawed beauty that is uniquely our own. Like wabi-sabi bowls we are perfectly imperfect. Remember the Ray Charles song titled *You Are So Beautiful to Me*? That's how I feel about each of you.

Here is what John O'Donohue writes about this, "One can only learn to see who one is when one learns to view oneself with the most intimate and forgiving compassion. Such a glimpse of one's essence can utterly rejuvenate a life and enable one to find the hidden wisdom in the beauty of the flaw."[19] We're all broken, patched and messy, but it's our flaws that make us unique, valuable, and yes, beautiful. Let's stop listening to the voices of perfection and welcome who we are and what we look like with open arms. We are all beautifully created.

GOING IN CIRCLES DOES NOT MEAN YOU'RE LOST

Being married to a pilot gave our family
lots of flying experience. For many years
we had access to a small airplane (think
Volkswagen of the sky) so we enjoyed
planning trips using that form of
transportation. How different the world
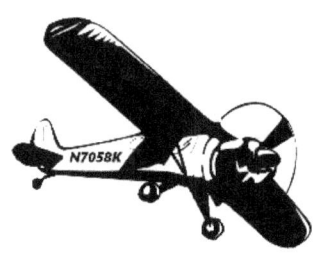
looks when our view is broadened. As a college student, one of Curt's
ways of earning money was to fly in different size circles while taking
aerial photos of resorts in northern Michigan and Wisconsin. The resorts
would purchase his pictures.

Later, as a family, flying in circles was fun when we wanted to enjoy a few
minutes looking at something especially interesting on the ground. While
in the air we could easily see weather conditions, and threatening
changes meant we would circle around and head back to the nearest
airport until the storm past. These circles did not represent being lost,
they represented enjoyment, productivity, and safety.

Circles are everywhere. Our human experience is often called "the circle
of life," which is reflected in many ancient beliefs and spiritual traditions.
In the circle of life, it's comforting to know that nothing ends without
something else beginning. We are cradled in that reassuring certainty.
The Oglala Sioux leader, Black Elk, taught "The power of the world
always moves in circles."[20] The repetition of changing seasons influences
our daily activities, and our journey from youth to old age, contain the
gift of lessons learned and wisdom earned. And, in those times when we
feel lost in our circle of life, we can choose different people and paths to
bring us home to ourselves.

Across the world there are historic and modern circular labyrinths. The labyrinth path takes walkers slowly back and forth into its center, and then returns them to the outside of the circle. This is a form of meditation that quiets the mind and calms the body, so we can center ourselves. Inside the circle the labyrinth path wonders back and forth, but people do not get lost. Taking a different path does not necessarily mean we're lost – we're just exploring our options. People can skip around the borders of the pathways, creating their own individual route, but they are still inside the circle. There is more than one path available for us to arrive at where we want to go.

Birds flying in thermal wind currents ride the air in a steady, relaxed, spiral path. They can glide this way for hours. Their flight is easy and unlabored. When humans go in circles, we immediately think we must be lost – and sometimes we are. When circumstances are difficult and life stress is high, our circles are needed the most, so we don't lose our way. We need our family circle to embrace us, and our circle of friends to listen. We need our professional colleague circle to reach out and our school circle to understand with support and encouragement. We need our medical community circle to be compassionate. All of these circles carry the potential to surround us with safety, love and belonging. With those three qualities we can, like the birds, glide in our spiral path resting unafraid in the currents of life that carry us.

One of my favorite circles is a hug. I don't care if there are two or twenty people participating, a hug feels so nourishing that I'm immediately renewed. It melts tension and says "I care" in a very personal way. Any one of the circles mentioned is enough to keep us from getting lost in the unexpected events of our lives.

Sarah Ban Breathnach writes the following about how she behaves when she gets lost in circumstances. "I've been too busy to write in my gratitude journal; I've begun dropping in my tracks because I'm unable to say "no"; I'm cranky because my house is cluttered and I can't find anything; I'm frazzled because I let myself forget that moments of solitude and meditation are necessary to center myself."[21] Any of that sound familiar? She then describes how she steps back, and starts over again to change how she reacts to her circumstances, so she finds a peaceful place in the circle of her day.

The spiral path to some is a philosophy, to others a spiritual journey that keeps us moving higher. From increasing height our view becomes broader and clearer. Yes, we're going in circles, but we are not lost. May your circle be filled with love, belonging, support, and safety.

HIDDEN TREASURE: OUR INNER RESOURCES

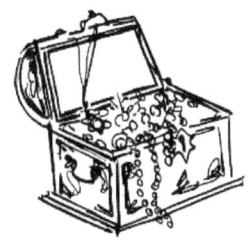

We all have times when we wonder if the buried treasure of our inner resources is actually there. When we're discouraged or depleted, our doubt in our abilities to cope may be especially strong as we wonder what happened to our skills, strength, and courage. It's important to know that, whatever is happening, our inner resources of love, guidance, healthy perspective, forgiveness, gratitude, and flexibility are always available.

Thich Nhat Hanh describes it this way, "We already are what we want to become. Even in our most difficult moments, everything that is good, true, beautiful is already there, within us and around us. We just have to live in such a way that allows it to be revealed."[22] We can be at peace with life. The more we use our inner resources, the stronger they become. So, let's go on a treasure hunt to remind ourselves of ways to find and build our inner resources.

Embracing our fears is easier said than done, but it does lead to treasure. Fear overrides what we really want; love, freedom to be ourselves, new experiences, and inner guidance. Acknowledging what is happening and accepting challenges will open the door to all of these, along with the gift of unexpected opportunities. When we welcome our challenges, instead of pushing them away, we move into trusting that whatever happens is perfectly orchestrated. This even includes when things are chaotic.

With patience and encouragement, we can take our toughest circumstance and cover it with acceptance and love, transforming it and us in the process. Psychologist Rick Hanson writes, "Mental resources like determination, self-worth, and kindness are what make us resilient: able to cope with adversity and push through challenges in the pursuit of opportunities."[23] Facing and embracing what scares us will reveal our hidden treasure and open the door to major breakthroughs.

Building inner resources happens when we spend time with confident, emotionally strong, productive people. These people inspire us and surround us with positive energy. We learn from their stories. Christine Northrup calls negative people "energy vampires"[24] and has written a book by that title. She clearly states that we need to step away from people who use and abuse us.

Our inner resources are strengthened when we spend time acknowledging our own past accomplishments, and the road blocks that were overcome in the process. This reaffirms that goals can be achieved despite difficulty. Even the people that look the most accomplished have had struggles. The difference lies in using and strengthening our inner resources.

Buried treasure is found when we embrace quiet time for reflection and gratitude. When we stop being busy and spend time with our thoughts and feelings, we get to know ourselves and have empathy for ourselves and others. Thich Nhat Hanh writes, "We have a tendency to think in terms of doing and not in terms of being. We think that when we are not doing anything we are wasting our time. But that is not true. Our time is first of all for us to be. To be what? To be alive, to be peaceful, to be joyful, to be loving. And that is what the world needs most."[25] When we declutter our minds, and take time to relax, we get in touch with our hidden treasures.

When we take responsibility for ourselves, we build inner resources. This means we do not make excuses when we make mistakes. We take responsibility for our actions, admit our mistakes, and forgive ourselves. This is hard and uncomfortable, but it's ultimately rewarding because it develops strength and resilience. Asking for help is also a sign of strength and can take many forms including counseling and therapy.

Ruth Nina Welsh writes, "But remember that while others can help you make the journey, only you can grasp the treasure. Only you can believe that you are special, a person of value and worth, with gifts and skills. Only you can claim your buried treasure."[26] Our inner resources are always ready and available. Let's claim the treasure that is ours.

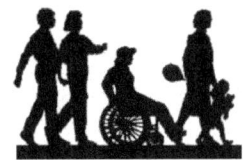

IN PRAISE OF SLOWNESS

Somehow the word slow and our culture don't seem to go together, and yet, my inner desire is to slow down. I read this quote by Thomas Merton, "To allow oneself to be carried away by a multitude of conflicting concerns, to surrender to too many demands, to commit oneself to too many projects, to want to help everyone in everything is to succumb to violence. The frenzy of the activist neutralizes his or her work for peace."[27] I was taken back by the strength of this statement concerning the importance of slowing down, honoring our limits, and the damage we do to ourselves if we don't. This message rings true.

Haven't we all had the experience of over committing ourselves because we didn't want to say "no"? Think about all the conversations we have about how busy we are – and we are! Sometimes it looks like a contest revealing who is busiest. Or, could we be afraid we'll miss something important so we pick up our pace, treat everything as if it were urgent, and overload our nervous system until we're overwhelmed. It doesn't matter how helpful the task or noble the intention if, in the process of giving ourselves away, we become unkind. When I'm overextended, I'm no longer able to be fully present for anyone or do any task well. I end up living out of reaction instead of reflection.

Sometimes life uses inconveniences to give us the message that we need to slow down. It can be waiting in line to make a purchase, dealing with a delay in travel, personal plans unraveling, or heavy traffic barely moving. And sometimes we are forced to slow down through illness. Cancer certainly slowed me down, and as I gradually recovered, I realized I didn't want to return to my previous "100mph Sylvia speed". I missed so much of life's magnificent scenery because I was trying to get wherever I wanted to go as fast as I could. John O'Donohue writes that, "In our obsession with instant access, we forget that the best things are discovered slowly."[28]

Each of us has a pace that works best for us – there is no one size fits all speed. The reward comes when we honor our limits with careful selection, so we can reclaim our centeredness, restore balance, experience inner calm, and slow ourselves into renewed health on all levels.

Cultivating slowness means making time for activities that defy acceleration like; yoga, reading, knitting, gardening, painting, kayaking, mediation, walking and chi gung. Carl Honore writes, "The great benefit of slowing down is reclaiming the time and tranquility to make meaningful connections--with people, with culture, with work, with nature, with our own bodies and minds"[29] This is exactly what I did (along with my husband and sister) a week ago.

At 8:15 am the three of us launched our kayaks at Round Island boat launch, and leisurely paddled into the Indian River Lagoon. Normally we plan the details of our outing, but this time we entered the water with no plan in place. We just wanted to see whatever there was to see. With relaxed strokes we began a pattern of paddling, and then quietly resting. Our focus on nature heightened our awareness of the wind song in the trees, bird melodies, and insect chirps. Then we noticed a group of pelicans still sleeping in their tree roost. While continuing to meander we saw a series of hunting osprey, kingfishers, blue herons, egrets, turkey vultures, anhinga, and cormorants. Fish were jumping and pelicans, the ones that had decided it wasn't too early for breakfast, were diving into the water with a spectacular splash, and emerging with a fish in their pouch. An adult and young manatee swam by, and then two dolphins appeared moving in unison. The sun played with tree shadow patterns on the water. We were so engrossed in our languid observations that two hours flew by before one of us checked a watch. The distance we covered was relatively small, but the dose of inner serenity was enormous. The restorative calmness and peace gained from our outing in nature is still with me – all I need to do is mentally put myself back in my kayak on the lagoon, and I am destressed and relaxed.

George Macdonald wrote, "Work is not always required...there is such a thing as sacred idleness, the cultivation of which is now fearfully neglected."[30] That is exactly what my kayak outing was – sacred, restorative idleness.

May we each take time for quiet reflection, discover and appreciate the gifts that slowness has to offer, and practice kindness to ourselves every day.

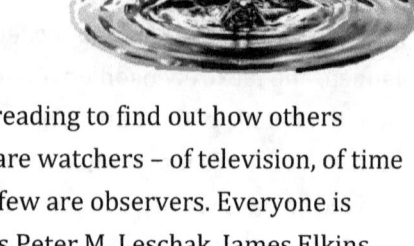

IS LOOKING THE SAME AS SEEING?

This question puzzled me so I began reading to find out how others viewed looking and seeing. "All of us are watchers – of television, of time clocks, of traffic on the freeway – but few are observers. Everyone is looking, not many are seeing"[31] writes Peter M. Leschak. James Elkins takes a look at this difference in his book "The Object Stares Back."[32] He suggests that looking sounds easy - we just turn our heads from side to side and take in what is going on around us.

Here's the difference. Looking is confined to being a form of general observation, detached from anything below the surface. Seeing uses our senses, intellect, and emotions which means our vision comes from within to embrace the whole subject. In James Elkins words, "Ultimately, seeing alters the thing that is seen and transforms the seer. Seeing is metamorphosis not mechanism."[33]

So, looking and seeing are not the same. We have a choice to look at our life experiences on the surface, or experience whatever shows up with our whole being. This distinction is especially helpful when we are dealing with some of life's challenges. Whether it is a serious illness, financial difficulties, job stress, or another car breakdown, looking keeps us on the surface reeling from circumstances. Seeing takes us below the surface where inner wisdom, peace, and patience reside. This is available to anyone who seeks the deeper meaning of our experiences.

This doesn't mean we deny the crisis, it means we look beneath the crisis. It was looking beneath the surface during my most serious challenges that opened my eyes to see the deeper meaning of my experience, along with the support that showed up in the most unexpected places that made each day a little easier. Like an archaeologist, we are rewarded when we dig deep.

We know that a lot goes on below the surface of the ground we walk on, or the ocean we swim in. It's also true that beneath the surface of our crisis are gifts of spiritual support, loving friendships, daily kindnesses, and needs met. This is where we see with our hearts the beauty and interconnectedness of all life. This is where we know beyond a doubt that no matter what is happening on the surface, we will be given everything we need exactly when we need it.

This kind of seeing takes practice and one effective way to start is through meditation. It's easier to pay attention to little nudges that indicate a deeper seeing when we're quiet. Any time our interest is aroused we need to listen, even if it doesn't make sense at the moment, or even if no one else thinks it's important, don't dismiss it. We all have antenna's that are working for us. So, tune into a question, a hunch, an observation, an idea, a pattern of connection, or a creative response. Let's pay attention and begin to notice what is going on beneath the surface. Let's make the most of every rich experience, especially the difficult challenges.

The eye that sees through the surface to read the heart and soul sees the uncovered promise that looking can't reveal. Seeing takes us beyond our labels and gives us an entrance into the remarkable world around and within us. Our life can be a feast so let's not hesitate, let's see deeply. Let's open our eyes and see our own metamorphosis. What will you discover today?

LEARNING TO BE FULLY PRESENT WITH OUR LIFE

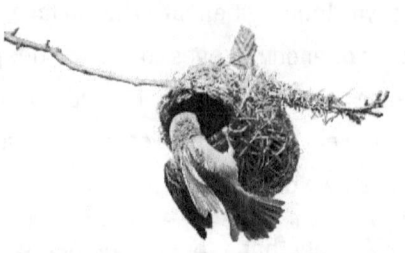

During my years of teaching high school, I practiced being fully present with my students so they knew they were heard and respected. As a wife I was conscious of being fully present with my husband when we needed to process what was happening between us, and as a mother I did the same with our two children. Looking back, I realize it was easier for me to be fully present with others, but harder for me to be fully present with myself. Once I understood that I couldn't give what I hadn't taken in, I began to practice being more fully present with myself.

Being present means creating awareness by paying attention to what is going on in our life from the big events, to small daily details. Since life is full of change, being willing to be flexible is essential as we continue to pay attention to each change. Being fully present creates a feeling of unity as mind, body, and spirit work in harmony. When we're truly present with our self, we learn about who we are more deeply with every life experience. If we intentionally focus on this moment, our mindfulness will help us go beneath the surface of what is happening, to the truth of what is happening. Without presence we miss this.

Since we' re surrounded by so much distraction and change, what can we do to keep ourselves living fully present? We can start by listening to our bodies. When we stop listening to what other people are saying and focus on what our body is saying, we can hear its wisdom. It might tell us to go outside for a walk, stay in bed and sleep in, see a doctor, take a hot bath, have a salad for lunch, meet a friend, or eat some chocolate (one of my favorite messages). The more we listen, the more present we become, until living in the moment becomes habit.

Another suggestion is listening to our feelings without analyzing or judging them. If we notice what comes up, we will discover what is getting in our way of being fully present with our life. If we feel anger, disappointment, fear, resentment, or worry, it is a message that we're either hanging on to yesterday, or projecting into the future. By experiencing those feelings and letting them go, we can move into a peaceful now, which is life enhancing. This is what presence is all about. In James Thurber's words, "Let us not look back in anger, nor forward in fear, but around in awareness."[34] This is an invitation to come home to our inner present self.

Learning to live without all the answers is easier said than done, but it too is a doorway to being more present. Wanting answers creates worries that lead to self-criticism and self-doubt about how we're going to handle certain situations. With courage and practice we can learn to surrender to knowing nothing, which makes us teachable. When we surrender to the guidance of our Higher Power, we no longer need to strain to find the answers because they will come without effort.

We become more present when we celebrate small joys. It's much easier to be present when we're completely focused on watching a bird build its nest, an orchid bud open, clouds changing shapes, or unexpectedly seeing a friend. Recently I was sent a gorgeous bouquet of flowers that were all in the bud stage. I am now relishing the pleasure of watching them slowly open. Every time I check on the flowers I'm completely in the moment with their scent, beauty, and serenity. Quiet meditation and yoga help keep us centered and aid in presence practice. It takes energy, patience, and dedication to make presence a priority.

Being fully present requires taking a break from the digital world. Necessary as that is, it is full of distractions, and if we aren't paying attention hours of our day are gone. Let's try eating lunch away from our computers, taking a walk without our phones, and listening to the sounds of nature without buds in our ears. A quiet mind is the doorway to presence.

Planning is important, but so is flowing, which means balance is needed. Lists are something I'm good at making and following, but if I become rigid, I miss the beauty of spontaneity. Being flexible allows us the opportunity to go with the flow, which is always much better than what I had planned. If we fight change by clinging to what we know, we miss out on the new opportunities change brings. In Eckhart Tolle's words, "Some changes seem negative at first glance, but they create the space for something new to arrive."[35] There's a gift of new energy and perspective in the unexpected. This is an opportunity to embrace what it has to offer which is living fully present.

As with any learning, this takes practice. The old adage, "Where attention goes, energy flows" is true, and we'll be amazed at what will change when we change our focus. We will move from victim to victor. One example would be the request that was made to stay home during COVID-19. Staying home can be seen as a prison or as a personal retreat — it's all a matter of attitude and attention. Learning to live in the present is a life changing journey that is empowering as we discover our own inner strength and resilience. Let's take Eckhart Tolle's advice, "Remember that the present is all you have. Make the 'now' the center of your life."[36]

LISTENING TO LIFE

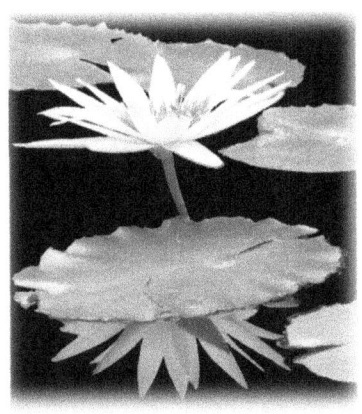

Our lives talk to us every day, but without listening we may miss its messages. Busyness, noise, smart phones and computers can dull our senses so we miss what life is trying to tell us. Learning to listen can take time because the guiding messages from within are often gentle and quiet. Parker Palmer said, "The soul speaks its truth only under quiet, inviting and trustworthy conditions."[37]

Life does not randomly happen. If we listen with awareness, we can usually see there are reasons behind events and emotions. If we are frustrated, angry, or fearful life is giving us a message. If we're sick, dealing with a broken relationship, or in a financial crisis there is a message. These are signs that something is not working and needs our attention. Being content, productive, and peaceful are all messages. Life is a mirror giving us an accurate reflection of our choices, habits and attitudes. It tells us how we're doing both inside and out.

John Kehoe writes about what he calls "The Sacred Wound."[38] This is the term he uses for the personal crisis we all have. He suggests a crisis happens because something wants to be noticed, or someone needs to be heard. Whatever form the crisis takes it shakes us to our core, so we examine our belief system and lifestyle. This is what makes a crisis so valuable – it invites us to see what changes are needed. Crisis can precede transformation which is why it is sacred. As an example, I didn't like my cancer diagnosis but, difficult as that was, I treasure what I learned during that time because it made me more authentic.

When we listen to what is happening in our life moment by moment, we enter a deeper place within us where we can respond with wisdom. This curbs knee jerk reactions which are usually counterproductive. Staying in the moment allows us to be more closely connected to our feelings, which are an important part of listening.

If you're like me, I need to constantly remind myself to stay in the moment. Here are a few things that help bring me back to the present. I do one thing at a time and focus completely on that activity whether it is combing my hair, driving the car, or listening to someone who's hurting. Taking several deep breaths is also helpful for calming and refocusing on the moment. Quiet meditation, no matter what time length, gathers scattered thoughts and lays them to rest. When I get quiet and ask for guidance there is always an answer. I also remind myself that every moment is precious, even the difficult ones, so I need to pay attention to them all.

A critical part of listening to our life is learning to trust our intuition. Intuition is part of the creative guidance that comes from our Higher Power. Messages from our intuition may arrive as a profound realization, or a grounded thought from deep within that provides a greater understanding of a subject, person, or life event. There can be physical sensations that go with this. For me a feeling of uneasiness tells me that I need to pay close attention to what is going on. A knot in my stomach is a signal that something is definitely wrong. A thought to quickly change what I'm doing means action is needed now.

Intuition saved my husband's life. He was in his car on 41st Street turning onto Indian River Boulevard. The light was already green as he approached the intersection, but a thought kept coming to him to slow down and not go into the intersection. He listened, and as he slowed a Cadillac SUV flew through the red light traveling at a high speed. Had Curt driven into the intersection, he would have been T- boned on the driver's side and killed. Sometimes intuition asks us to defy logical reasoning. He said he heard his guardian angel. I'm deeply grateful he listened.

Our life is talking to us every minute of every day. Messages come when we're having a conversation, driving, dealing with a problem at work, viewing art, relaxing with music, preparing a meal, taking a walk or playing with our pets. The list is endless. Honing our listening skills adds to the quality of each moment, because through listening we embark on the journey of identifying our true desires, and discovering who we were created to be. This is how author Fredrick Buechner sums this up, "Listen to your life. See it for the fathomless mystery it is. In the boredom and pain of it no less than in the excitement and gladness: Touch, taste, smell your way to the holy and hidden heart of it because in the last analysis all moments are key moments......listen to your life."[39]

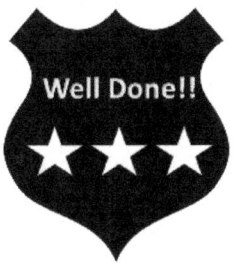

THANKING OURSELVES

Many of us grew up with the parental admonition to say "thank you" when receiving a kindness. In turn, we instruct our children to do the same. To stop there leaves out something important – thanking ourselves and our bodies for what we accomplish each day; for what we have been through; for the continuing functions of our mind and bodies. When was the last time you stopped to thank yourself for the incredible person you are, and your body for the amazing job it does for you each day? We show love and appreciation to those around us, but we often forget to do the same for ourselves. Here are a few suggestions for getting started.

91

Let's thank ourselves, along with our Higher Power, for the courage and strength everyday living requires. Whether it's relationships, health, finances, jobs, or parenting, we all have challenging situations we must deal with regularly. As the details of each day evolve, we evaluate our resources, and manage them to the best of our ability. If we're ill and in the middle of treatment, it's important to stop and thank ourselves for hanging in there, and doing what needs to be done. Courage shows itself in many ways. Mary Anne Radmacher writes, "Courage doesn't always roar. Sometimes courage is the quiet voice at the end of the day saying, I will try again tomorrow."[40] Often we are stronger than we know, and that deserves an affirmation.

Let's thank ourselves for our own unique beauty that comes from being authentic. When we live our life with integrity, we shine our light wherever we go, becoming a path finder for others. Doing what we know to be right, even though no one is looking, is being authentic and deserves a "well done." Taking care of our bodies by nurturing them on all levels (physical, spiritual, mental, emotional) enhances our inner beauty by affirming who we were born to be, and our outer beauty by putting a glow in our skin, a shine in our eyes, and a smile on our face.

Let's thank ourselves for being brave enough to listen to our heart and intuition, which is the voice of our Higher Power. Albert Einstein wrote, "The intuitive mind is a sacred gift and the rational mind is a faithful servant. We have created a society that honors the servant and has forgotten the gift."[41] Every time we ignore the loud voices around us, and listen to the quiet voice within, we honor our spiritually guided intuition. It is bold and brave to live in alignment with our inner wisdom. This deserves acknowledgement.

Let's thank ourselves for our thirst for growth. When we value our experiences as a tool for growth, we open ourselves to life changing lessons found even in the most difficult circumstances. Like an alchemist, we take every life interaction and turn it into new found wisdom. Turning wounds into wisdom deserves a big "well done."

Let's thank ourselves for practicing forgiveness with the help of our Higher Power. We know that holding onto grudges, anger, and resentment, is toxic for us and everyone around us. Forgiving releases us from this damage, enhances physical and mental health, and improves all our relationships. The act of forgiving releases us from living in negativity. Every time we practice forgiveness, we can choose to appreciate the miracle that has just happened.

Let's thank ourselves for actively using our sense of humor. Even the most difficult situations can feel less stressful when we practice appropriate humor. When used with sensitivity humor can lighten a funeral service, bring a smile to a hospital room, soften behavior corrections, or diffuse conflict. Every time we do this, we lighten up the situation and boost the spirits of the people around us.

Let's thank our bodies for the service they do for us each day. During a recent massage I thought about all the things my feet do for me without getting any acknowledgement. Then I began to think about the rest of my body that I often take for granted, until something breaks down. The incredible inner and outer workings of our bodies are amazing, and deserve love and appreciation for the miracle of their daily performance.

Today, take time to thank yourself for the unique person you are, with all your courage, strength, inner listening, commitment to love, messy imperfections, and daily accomplishments. Take time to acknowledge what's been learned over the years, and what's been done with what was learned. If this sounds too hard, choose one thing to appreciate and honor about yourself today. It's time to give yourself the credit you deserve!

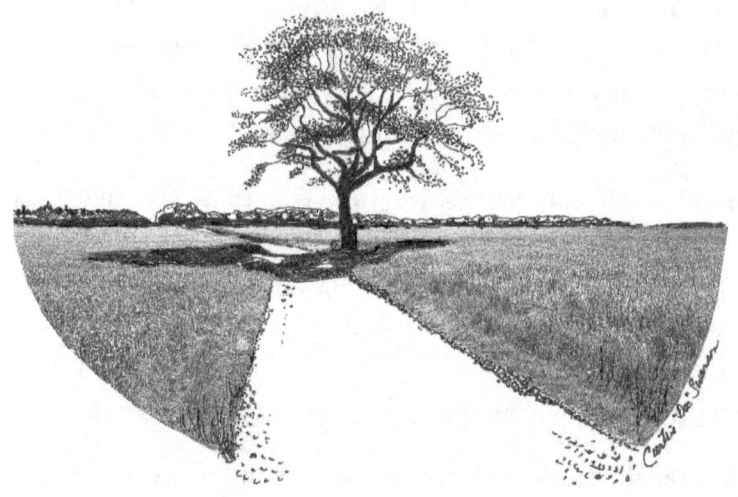

Chapter 4 - Self-Care

CHAOS, NOISE, & GRIT

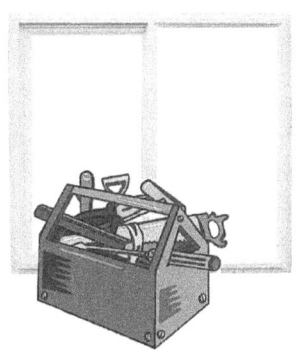

Everything at my condo is in such disarray that I have fled to my sister's quiet house. Our windows were outdated and needed to be replaced, so the process began yesterday when the new windows were delivered. Installing hurricane windows is a noisy process but I didn't realize the full extent of the noise until air drills and power saws were singing a duet. It's ear piercing and goes on all day!

Furniture needed to be rearranged in every room, so all the pieces were pushed together to make space for our 6-man crew (one woman did arrive to make sure the men were doing what they were supposed to do). Everyone commented on what perfect weather we were having for a large, mostly outdoor project.

The breeze was wonderful until we realized the wind was blowing cement grit (from their drilling) everywhere inside our condo; the furniture, lamp shades, book shelves, blinds, carpet, computer, kitchen counters, stove, sofas, tables and chairs. A major cleaning will be needed which won't start until the installers are finished. This morning we brought out every sheet we own and covered as much as possible to eliminate adding more grit. More laundry but less grit.

My husband, the engineer, was watching the design of the new windows and the system of replacement with enjoyment. He seemed to be at ease with the whole process, but the chaos, noise, and grit challenged my limits. For my sanity's sake I had to escape! I'm reminded of this quote from Melody Beattie that says, "Few situations are bettered by going berserk."[1] Going berserk from the noise was a definite possibility, and the only way to avoid it was by honoring my limits and moving into healthy self-compassion. That meant leaving the installation scene.

On the other side of town, my sister and her three cats offered a welcome oasis of tranquility and quiet. Curt joined us for lunch and late afternoon sipping time. We all need a safe shelter when chaos, noise and grit take over. Perspective (chaos, noise and grit won't last forever) and calmness (my emotional reaction) are extremely valuable when navigating a difficult situation. Both anxiety and calmness are contagious, so the question according to Brené Brown is, "Do we want to infect people with more anxiety, or heal ourselves and the people around us with calm?"[2]

If we are kind to ourselves, we create a reservoir of caring compassion, which means our own needs are met and we have more to offer others. Here is what Christopher K. Germer says about the importance of self-compassion, "A moment of self-compassion can change your entire day. A string of such moments can change the course of your life."[3] The only way I could survive the installation process, and take care of myself, was to leave the site and seek a calm, quiet place.

I'm grateful for the new windows and the work crew that made it possible as well as having what we need to clean the house. What I'm most grateful for is Curt's understanding encouragement to seek a quiet shelter. My sanity is now intact and flourishing. Whenever we're faced with any form of chaos, noise, or grit, let's remind ourselves that now is the time for self-care and compassion. We are worthy and deserving!

COMFORTING OURSELVES WHEN WE'RE MOST UNCOMFORTABLE

Life gives us numerous opportunities to be uncomfortable in an intense

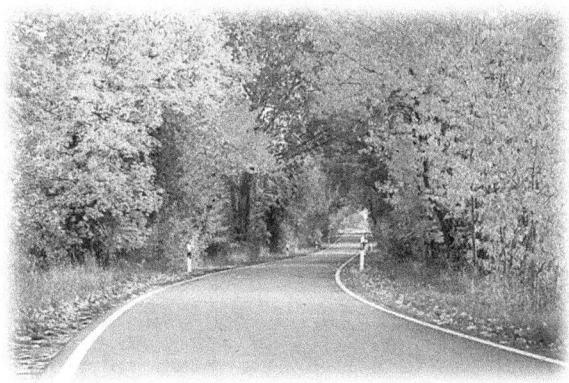

way we may not have experienced before. Along with this, we are also given an opportunity to dig deep into our inner resources, and discover more courage and strength than we thought we had. There is comfort in recognizing the enormous potential we have to work our way through a crisis and emerge wiser, and better able to handle the next challenge.

Any challenge usually produces a whole gamut of emotions from shocked, overwhelmed, and heavy-hearted to hopeful, peaceful and calm. We can have comfortable and uncomfortable emotions at the same time. Jonatan Martensson writes, "Feelings are much like waves, we can't stop them from coming but we can choose which ones to surf."[4]

Embracing our vulnerability and comforting ourselves lessens tension and allows calmness, humor, nature, play, food, music, meditation, and gratitude to alter attitudes and work their peaceful magic. Humor comforts and produces a hearty laugh that lightens up everything. Wherever you find humor pass it on so others can destress through laughter.

Anytime we are dealing with something serious we need more than ever to enjoy the comfort of play. Gather whoever you live with and together make up wonderfully ridiculous stories, passing the storytelling around the circle. Those living alone can still be creative with their own story that is shared with neighbors or mailed to family. We can relive embarrassing moments (admit it – we all have them), dance in our living room, get out the card and board games, and promote general silliness. Forget what anyone else may think, this is the time to be whimsical and spontaneous.

We can get out your walking shoes and head out into nature for comfort. Feel the breeze in our hair, watch the wind in the trees, look for what flowers are blooming, and listen to bird song. Breathe that fresh air in deeply. I love checking up on our resident Sandhill Cranes and catching a glimpse of an Armadillo. It promotes a connection with the world. Take the opportunity to wave at neighbors and exchange news. If walking isn't an option sit on your porch and enjoy whatever the day brings.

Everyone has their own list of comfort foods. Get out your favorite recipes and cook up a batch of whatever brings you pleasure. Take time to savor that morning cup of coffee or tea. If our usual ingredients aren't available let's make up new favorites with everyone helping in the kitchen. There is both enjoyment and solace in good food – and it doesn't all have to be healthy. Treats are needed too.

Whatever your taste in music, it can be a balm to a weary heart. Play that favorite opera, symphony, rock and roll band, or currently enjoyed artist. Put on your comfort clothes with bright colors (this is not the time for black!), and sing along. Recently someone posted on Facebook a group of artists who came together to sing "What the World Needs Now Is Love Sweet Love"[5] and it brought me to tears. It was beautifully done and the message was timely. Another Facebook posting was a choir singing the hymn, "It Is Well With My Soul" and "I Have Peace Like A River" which also brought me to tears it was so comforting. Pick your genre and let it calm your thoughts and sooth your soul. There's also deep comfort in exercising your faith in a Higher Power and meditating or praying in whatever way works best for you.

Keeping in touch with friends and family is essential so let's use whatever resources we have to do that. The comfort we give and receive from the people we love helps to keep us balanced. This is where gratitude blooms, and clarity is enhanced. Your grocery store, your neighborhood, the internet is full of beautiful stories of generosity that offer comfort and reassurance of the overflowing kindness that is at the center of our hearts. When we focus on gratitude we change the energy around us, and discomfort and worry fade, allowing love to transform our experience into a uniting, supporting, sacred event. Let's be patient with the people around us, let go of our worries, and relax into nurturing comfort. In the words of Winnie The Pooh, "You are braver than you believe, stronger than you seem, and smarter than you think."[6]

CULTIVATING SELF-COMPASSION

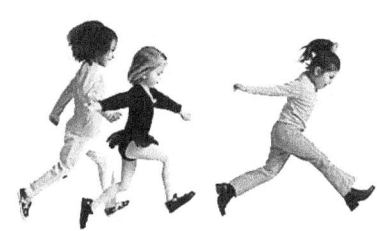

"Love and compassion are necessities, not luxuries. Without them humanity cannot survive."[7] (Dalai Lama) Self-compassion isn't about being selfish or arrogant; it's about treating our bodies with gentleness, kindness, empathy, and acceptance. It's about loving ourselves with the compassion we often give others, but at times deny ourselves. Whenever we go through an unexpected event, let's acknowledge our emotions without guilt or judgement. It's important to be gentle with our feelings. We may find ourself in a situation we aren't prepared for, so this is the time self-compassion is most needed.

Let's remember self-compassion isn't shallow or abstract, it's a well-researched and acknowledged survival tool. So, let's look at this tool. Here are a few suggestions for cultivating self-compassion. First let's accept things just as they are and stop forcing life to do our bidding. When we stop struggling against trying to make life be what we want it to be, and just relax into accepting what we have no control over, an incredible burden is lifted and we experience peace and grace.

Our self-talk is another tool to use for self-compassion. Negative self-talk can easily pollute our day and, if you're like me, some days I am my own worst critic. This is the opposite of self-compassion. A shift to positive self-talk invites empowerment, encouragement and lowered stress. Now that's a good motivator for change.

Cultivating patience, with an attitude of being gentle with ourselves, also fosters self-compassion. We honor our limits. The more rigid our expectations, the more frustrated and angrier we'll be if this doesn't blend with what we can realistically do right now. If we've discovered we're not up for that new project, let's let it go. Self-compassion accepts that what we want to happen will happen when the time is right.

Self-compassion involves forgiving ourselves when mistakes happen. We all make them, and chances are we'll make more. Mistakes are part of how we learn and grow as humans. If we let our failures define us, we become stuck in an agonizing place. Let's release ourselves from guilt with forgiveness. It's important to feel free to try new activities so we can discover what we are capable of doing.

Gratitude enhances self-compassion. Believing that the Universe wants us to thrive will make it easier to find the resources we need. I'm grateful for whatever food there is in the grocery (my favorite brands no longer matter), mail that gets delivered, humor showing up on Facebook. I think we are all thankful for the loving people we have in our lives, but let's also be grateful for ourselves and how far we've come. Gratitude is a channel for compassion.

Part of cultivating self-compassion is keeping positive people around us. People who put us down are not friends and will bring out the worst in us. Supportive, encouraging people will bring out our best. Let's spend time with friends who enjoy playing. It's important to loosen up and celebrate ourselves. Play releases endorphins which makes us feel good all over, and who doesn't need more of that. Saying "no" to anything that isn't right for us honors our own needs, and releases us from the "people pleasing club". Honoring the time we need to give to our self is having compassion for our self.

Every day there is an opportunity for self-compassion. In the words of Christopher Germer, "A moment of self-compassion can change your entire day. A string of such moments can change the course of your life."[8]

FRAGILE – HANDLE WITH LOVING CARE

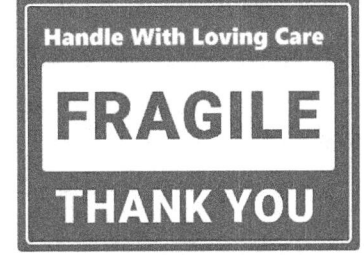

Handing me the phone my husband said, "It's the dermatologist's office."
As I listened, the nurse informed me that the biopsy on my leg showed severe stage pre-cancer tissue with horizontal spreading roots. Surgery to remove it needed to be scheduled. A referral to a plastic surgeon of my choice would be made. My first thought was I didn't want to handle one more, even small, thing right now. My second thought was I need to love myself. I was feeling fragile.

Feeling fragile is not a sign of weakness, it's a sign of sensitivity to what is happening in our lives. When we're fragile we experience what is happening with an intensity that can lead to feeling overwhelmed. Most of us have experienced that. We can use our fragileness to become victims threatened by circumstances, and react by building protective walls around ourselves. Or we can choose to stay calm, find our balance, validate our self-worth, and love ourselves through the challenging situation.

Combining healthy self-care with mindfulness will help us navigate those times of feeling fragile. This has everything to do with loving ourselves. Jen Underwood writes, "See the places that are tender within you, and move carefully around them. Show them love and kindness. Erase the judgement. And move very, very, slowly."⁹ It's time to give ourselves permission to thoughtfully determine what it is we want or need in this given moment. And then, without guilt, give ourselves permission to do just that. This creates a beautiful oasis of gentle self-care that is nurturing.

One of the best ways to love our fragile selves is to be grateful for who we are and what we have right now. With gratitude we can value ourselves without validation from anyone else, and we can honor being true to ourselves over being perfect. Gratitude can turn pain and frustration into a motivator, and acknowledges that we are in control of the way we look at our life. Through the eyes of gratitude, we can see the presence of the Divine in everything that happens, and we know we are being handled with loving care whatever the circumstances.

We handle ourselves with loving care when we embrace what is. One of the greatest presents we can give ourselves is to pay close attention to our life as we're living it. So much is lost when we pay attention to the distraction we carry; such as a mobile phone in the palm of our hand. If we can be consistently present, we experience the beauty and depth of each moment. Life is about what happens between now and our next breath and, whatever that holds, acceptance is the door that brings in grace. It's out of acceptance that the solution arises.

We especially need to forgive ourselves for past mistakes when we're feeling fragile. The light of forgiveness banishes our dark places so we can let go of the past. In Eckhart Tolle's words, "Sometimes letting things go is an act of far greater power than defending or hanging on."[10] Once we do this act, we can start making needed changes. Then we can move away from things that drain us, and move toward what nourishes and fulfills us.

Doing what makes us happy is another way of handling ourselves with loving care. When we do things we care about we're nurtured and refreshed. Kayaking is something I enjoy doing so, even though there is work involved in organizing supplies, loading and unloading and washing them down after use, I have a grateful tiredness. The quiet time out on the water is worth the effort. Doing things that make us happy is loving self-care.

We handle ourselves with loving care when we're honest with ourselves about everything. This means expressing our pain without reckless, unchecked behavior. It means comforting ourselves when we're anxious and listening to our intuition when we're decision making. When we want to try something new we don't let not knowing how it will turn out keep us from beginning something new. Marc Chernoff writes, "When we act uncertainty chases us out into the open where opportunity awaits."[11] Let's believe in our abilities and acknowledge our skills. When we're having a fragile moment, let's remember that the best way to navigate rough waters is to handle ourselves with loving care.

HELLO DAY – WHAT IS IT I NEED TO KNOW?

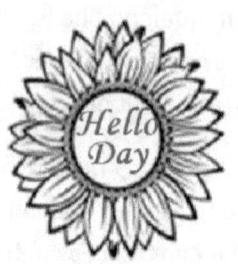

There are so many ways to greet a new day,
and how we choose to do it affects our
experience of the day's events. My husband
and I had an unplanned experiment involving starting the day in two
different ways. One morning we got up, grabbed our phones and began
checking the news. At the breakfast table all we could talk about was how
awful the news was, and by the end of the meal we were both distraught
and crabby. It took most of the day to eliminate that negative energy. The
decision was made not to do that again.

The next morning, we left our phones alone, picked up our favorite book
of spiritual poetry and read to each other. We felt energized, uplifted and
positive about the day, and this was reflected in our breakfast
conversation. The tone of the whole day was set by how we began the
day. It was a valuable lesson to both of us in setting clear intentions when
we welcome a fresh day. Intentions reflect what is most important to us.
The intention we set was to begin the day with self-care and kindness so
that could flow throughout the day

What we need to know is that intention is like a seed that is nourished by
our attention – the more attention it receives, the more it flourishes.
What kind of intentional seeds do we want to nurture? One that I want to
nurture is gratitude. When I first wake up, I think about what I'm grateful
for and say a prayer of thanks. After nourishing the seed of gratitude at
the beginning of the day, I continue to experience gratitude throughout
the day.

If we set the intention that we're going to trust that what we need
throughout the day will be provided, we'll have a calmness within us so

life's little surprises, like a dead car battery or the phone call that brings difficult news, won't send us into a tailspin. That's because we're leaning into trust. Trust that says "All will be well."

If the intention of taking good care of our bodies is chosen, we can do gentle stretches after getting out of bed, drink a glass of water and select a healthy breakfast. With the intention of being an attentive listener we will do less talking and learn more about the people around us. Choosing to remain true to ourself throughout the day will clarify decision making. We can choose to do acts of kindness which enhance both the giver and the receiver. Intentions can be courage, compassion, finishing a project or being completely present with the people around us.

What we need to know is that morning routines are important, but no one routine works for everyone. It can be fun to discover what works for our particular needs. These choices will ground us so we feel ready to meet a new day. It's this early morning focus that sets the pattern for the day rather than the day being in charge of us. So, let's hug our kids, pets or spouse, and take a moment for meditation, prayer or journaling to prepare us for the day ahead.

The idea is to integrate into welcoming the day whatever works best for each of us so we begin the day well. If we keep it simple, with clear intentions, our whole day will improve. This doesn't mean difficult things won't happen, it means we will be better able to handle them. By doing this we gain clarity, calmness and increased confidence in handling whatever happens. Let's say hello to our day with thoughtfulness and the intention to start the day the best way possible.

HONORING OUR FEELINGS

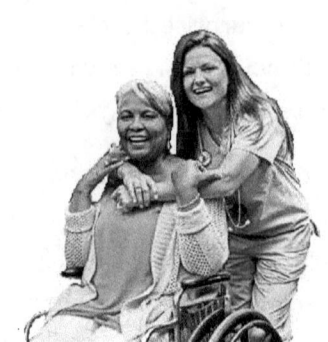

As human beings we experience an
array of feelings ranging from simple
to complex. Feelings are not valid or
invalid; good or bad; they simply are
part of life and you. When we are
brave enough to slow down and mindfully listen, our feelings surface and
show us their gifts. The key is to own what we are feeling, experience it
fully, release it, and acknowledge its gift. The more we do this, the better
we feel about ourselves and what caused those feelings.

Sometimes it's hard to put a name on what we're feeling. All we know is
that we have a heavy heart. Well-meaning people can suggest that an
incident we are trying to process isn't a big deal, advising us to get life
into perspective. It is never helpful to tell someone how they should feel
about an event in their life. If that happens, we need to remind ourselves
that what we are feeling is real and valid.

Sometimes we know right away what feeling is being triggered, and
we're afraid to let it show. Honoring our feelings means that when we are
mourning a loss, we don't need to pretend we're not struggling. Our
struggle is real. When negotiating a major life change, we don't need to
hide our insecurity. When managing a depleting illness, we need to turn
personal criticism into compassion for ourselves. When we have been
disrespected, betrayed, or violated in any way, feelings of anger and a
need to be understood are important. It doesn't matter what is significant
or insignificant to anyone else, our feelings deserve respect.

Rushing, over doing, over giving, over eating, and over performing are
habits that keep us from being in touch with our emotions. The more
present we are with our feeling reality, the more we benefit. Author

Linda Popov writes, "The key is to give yourself permission to experience your feelings, own them, then release them. When you do this, you will emerge into a lighter, more vital place. I promise you, you will feel more alive and your relationships will benefit from your increased vitality."[12]

When we have processed our feelings, we need to give them a healthy release. Talking it out with a trusted friend can be therapeutic. A feeling journal is an excellent way to clarify what is happening. Creating art, music, or poetry is a helpful release as well as long walks in nature. Treat yourself to what makes you feel good; a long hot bubble bath, a favorite beverage, a long read in your favorite relaxing place, watch a movie, get a massage, talk to a supportive friend, and above all be kind and gentle with yourself.

For those times when life is so overwhelmingly difficult and we are angry, we can be creative in releasing anger. I've used pillow pounding, vigorous stone throwing into a lake (not at people), and driving to an isolated corner of a park to scream (with the windows up) until I felt relieved. This is much better than yelling at our families or kicking the dog. And remember, there's nothing like a good nose reddening, puffy eyed, Kleenex drenching cry. Exercising vigorously is another way to release pent up feelings with the added advantage of burning extra calories. A dance instructor shared the advantages of dancing as therapy. The instructor freely admitted to dancing around his house with his movements reflecting his feelings. If our dancing rendition looks more like stomping then dancing, it doesn't matter. We're discharging our anger and the benefit is still there.

By having the courage to honor our feelings, we open ourselves to the gifts available through our increased understanding of emotions. We pick up on subtle details of the day that might otherwise have slid by from lack of attention; the sun shining through a branch outside a window; the smile on the face of an elder; the laughter of a child at play; the way hot chocolate smells before it's even tasted. We act instead of react because we are in tune with how we are feeling.

Our emotional center is a valuable part of us carrying with it the gift of increased health and wholeness. Through honoring our feelings, we can learn to more fully love our self and others, and be loved in return. That sounds like a productive way to begin each day.

KNOWING WHEN TO QUIT

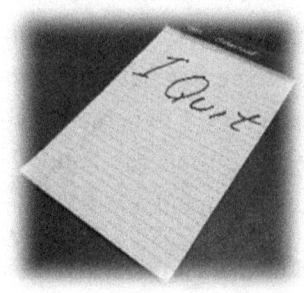

Haven't we all made the decision, at some point in time, to stop doing what no longer felt right? It can be an act of emancipation that encourages a step toward a more satisfying life. It can also be a surprise to the people around us causing some to be distressed and others envious.

The New York Times had a feature section that told the stories of nineteen people who had said "I quit!" to a variety of activities.[13] It takes courage to draw a line and say no to toxic relationships, unwanted products, doctors and treatment plans not in our best interest, foods that harm our bodies, or unreasonable demands from anyone, especially the people we love. I'd like to share a few of these stories so we can all be more empowered to know when the most nourishing choice is to walk away.

Veronica Chambers is a woman of color who was working for a magazine. Her white supervisor told her "... a black woman will never have my job." However, her supervisor used all of Veronica's ideas to revamp the magazine. She stuck with the job hoping she could advance. On a long weekend vacation with her husband and daughter, she carefully thought through her job scenario, and by the end of the weekend she knew she had to quit her job to keep her sanity.

What came next for her was writing four New York Times best sellers, two James Beard awards, and having one of her novels turned into a movie. She taught at Stanford University and Smith College. And she finally had more time to spend with her daughter. In Veronica's words, "When you're constantly shown to the back of the career bus, quitting what looks like a good job can be a vital moment of reclaiming the self-esteem that unlocks a world of possibility."[14]

Anna Dubenko quit graduate school when she knew it wasn't working for her. In her words, "Quitting graduate school was the hardest thing I've ever done – and I've given birth without an epidural."[15] Difficult as it was, she is now free to pursue what she truly desires. Lisa Wells quit her smartphone when she found herself paying more attention to her phone than to the people most important in her life.[16] Len Schreiner quit the priesthood when he fell in love.[17]

John Hogue felt conflicted about his consumerism habits, and decided to quit buying things thoughtlessly. In his words, "Not buying things has freed me to have more time, space and energy for relationships with others – including God."[18] Iva Dixit quit her elaborate skin-care routine after deciding the only person she needed to please was herself.[19] Nathan Pemberton quit his evangelical church when the church stopped listening to God and started telling God what to do.[20]

Eckhart Tolle wrote, "Awareness is the greatest agent for change."[21] When I read that quote, I began thinking of the times in my life that I became aware of the need for change. During an illness I went to a doctor who gave me a diagnosis and a prescription. I had a bad reaction to the drug, but the doctor blew it off. Knowing I was in the wrong place I quit that medical practice and found myself a doctor who cared. I've quit coloring my hair and embraced every grey hair on my head.

Whatever our challenges are, it's important to know when we have reached our limit and need to walk away. We have the power to manage our lives with mindfulness and clarity, so our choices nourish and support us. Let's support each other as we all take steps to free ourselves from what we need to quit doing, so we can live the life we truly want to live.

NOPE – NOT DOING THAT   *Nope Nope Nope*

If we're into people pleasing, "no" is one of the hardest words to say. For our own health and wellbeing, we need to think carefully and listen with the "ears of our heart" for what is right for us. Disappointing other people is far better than running ourself into a state of exhaustion or denying what we hold dear. Even though it isn't easy, personal experience tells me this essential.

A while back a friend asked me to join a social activity I had no interest in. To be true to myself I thanked her for the invitation but declined coming. There was an organization I considered joining that required a pledge be spoken out loud. The pledge asked me to do things I didn't believe in and couldn't support, so I said "no." I have said no to doctors who did not have my best interest in mind, and counselors who had their own agenda and weren't interested in why I was there. I've also given in to the pressure of saying "yes" and regrated it later.

Time is precious to all of us so let's learn how to stand up for ourselves. Alice Boyes Ph.D. wrote an article titled, "How to Recognize When You Don't Have to Do Something"[22] suggesting that sometimes we fail to see we don't need to say yes. It can happen when others make a request of us and is especially hard if it's family or close friends. They can be more than persuasive; they can be coercive and manipulative. Anyone who knows us well can push our guilt button or invoke fear, but doing a request out of guilt or fear is unhealthy for everyone involved. This is where we protect ourself with boundaries and a "no" – even if it makes someone else unhappy. People pleasing is a tough way to live because it can deplete our inner resources.

Boyes suggests we can be harder on ourself than other people are when we tell ourself we need to do more than is healthy or necessary. Much as I love crossing things off my to do list, I also know balance is the key to taking care of myself. What is most important is our priorities, so if we value inclusion, we will not participate in organizations that are exclusive. Justice, the environment, equality, respect, health, and financial stability are a few other priorities that guide our choice of saying "yes" or "no."

"Part of psychological health is feeling empowered and being able to act in our own best interests even when we feel intimidated. In most cases, our actions should be driven by our values rather than by trying to avoid temporary negative emotions."[23] (Boyes)

Let's be empowered for the sake of our wallet which means saying "no" to repeated loan requests, expensive restaurants or one to many charities. We say "no" to protect our time which is precious. And we say "no" to protect our sanity.

We can practice courtesy and assertiveness when we say "no" and we don't need to make excuses. If our "no" is not accepted by someone we considered a friend then they are being disrespectful. If the issue is truly important to us, we stand firm, even when the other person is uncomfortable. People pleasing doesn't create the intimacy we crave so we end up frustrated and disappointed. When we're clear on what is and isn't our job, we can avoid burnout, too.

 Susan Biali Haas M.D. writes, "Though it feels like we're avoiding unpleasant consequences by bending to the needs of others, things are sure to get worse, not better, in our relationships, life and even health if we don't learn to live within our own boundaries."[24] Let's have the courage to say, "Nope – not doing that" when needed for our own wellbeing. The ears of our heart are an accurate guide and practice will enhance our comfort. We're not being selfish – we're taking care of ourself.

OUR BODIES ARE LISTENING

When fibromyalgia first arrived, it came on so strong that I was taken by surprise and completely overwhelmed. What started as a shoulder injury, turned into a level of full body pain I had never before experienced. I had no idea what was happening, and I was angry about what this was doing to my life. I was teaching high school full time, (using up all my sick days), parenting 2 college students, and taking continuing education classes. After an assortment of doctors, I finally had my diagnosis, and could begin appropriate therapies. Wanting to help myself as much as possible I read books, sought advice, consulted complementary medical resources, and practiced meditation. It was through meditation that I received the message that I needed to love myself, and let go of my anger. My prolonged anger was hurting me.

Meditation enhances communication between mind and body. Cleve Backster[25] is a researcher who spent 36 years studying communication in plant, animal, and human cells. The results of his work show that we experience emotions even at the cellular level. When we treat ourselves with compassion and kindness, our bodies receive that emotional message and use this positive energy for health improvement. When we talk to ourselves in a harsh, self-critical way we send our stress hormones soaring, aggravate inflammation, and become more susceptible to illness.

Our bodies are always listening and responding to every message we give them. Once I realized what was possible, I began my own program of letting go of anger, and embracing myself with love. What a difference that made!

Gradually I began improving mentally, emotionally, spiritually. It felt so good to stop being angry because life wasn't the way I wanted it to be, and focus on giving myself tender, loving, care. Then I began to improve physically, and learned to become patient with the process I was in. I was healing from the inside out. One by one I let go of all the pills, the TENS machine, and medical professionals who were not helpful. Today I still have fibromyalgia, but it is minor instead of major. I am now in the habit of monitoring the messages I give my body because the connection is so clear. My well-being depends on it.

This is one reason why being around positive people is so important. Masaro Emoto writes, "If you fill your heart with love and gratitude, you will find yourself surrounded by so much you can love that you can feel grateful for, and you can even get closer to the life of health and happiness that you seek. But what will happen if you emit signals of hate, dissatisfaction, and sadness? Then you will probably find yourself in a situation that makes you hateful, dissatisfied, and sad."[26] The choice is ours.

Another way our bodies listen is through music. Sometimes we listen without being fully aware of its impact. Don Campbell, in his book The Mozart Effect writes, "In an instant music can uplift our soul. It awakens

113

within us the spirit of prayer, compassion, and love. It clears our minds and has been known to make us smarter. Music can dance and sing our blues away. It conjures up memories of lost lovers or deceased friends. It lets the child in us play, the monk in us to pray, the cowgirl in us to line dance, the hero in us surmount all obstacles. It helps the stroke patient find language and expression."[27]

Today there is healing music created to match the personal vibrations of our bodies. I know this works because I have used this kind of music in my journey through fibromyalgia, back surgery, and cancer. Since our bodies are listening, what do we really want them to hear? Loud, harsh, angry music is not helpful. Now we have even more reason to enjoy our favorite positive music - our bodies are listening.

Isn't it helpful to know we are in charge of the messages we give our bodies? Let's take our power of choice and select the messages we need today. And let's be sure to share encouraging, affirming messages with all who need them. May your body rejoice in this day because every cell is responding to your loving messages.

RADICAL ACCEPTANCE

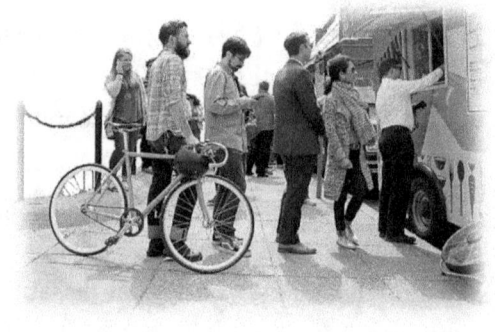

What does it mean to radically accept something? Does it mean that we give up on any possibility of change and become a doormat? Definitely not – it is anything but passive. It's a conscious choice that puts us in the best position to accept ourself, others and life completely with mind, body and spirit. It's accepting life on its terms, and acknowledging the parts that can't be changed. What we can't change becomes what allows us to participate in radical acceptance, and creative decision making.

We can practice acceptance in smaller situations such as rain on the day we wanted to go to the beach, heavy traffic, or a long wait in a doctor's office. Acceptance is like a muscle – the more we use it the stronger it gets. I got some practice the other day when, after not buying shoes for two years, I ordered a pair I thought would be the color I needed only to discover they weren't. Really!! The rain, cancelled plans, long waits and shoe color were all items that couldn't be changed, but they definitely don't represent a crisis. Practicing in the small areas prepares us for life's bigger challenges.

COVID-19, a cancer diagnosis (it took me a while to accept mine), an unfaithful spouse, job loss, or the passing of a loved one all significantly impact our life. Therapist Andrew Harris writes, "Completely and totally accepting this fact is still challenging and painful, but focusing on what we can control versus what we cannot, can be liberating. It frees up all of the energy we were using to fight reality, and helps us use it to focus on how we can effectively cope with the situation and take care of ourselves."[28] Let's allow ourself to feel sadness and grief when major things happen so we can transition to clearer vision. It's acceptance that frees us to see more options.

How do we live radical acceptance? First, we don't accept things we can change. We don't accept abuse, manipulation, or inappropriate behavior from our boss at the workplace. Social injustices, cruelty in any form, spreading misinformation and disrespectful behavior are not acceptable. Karyn Hall Ph.D. offers this advice, "If we have a problem we can solve, then that is the first option. If you can't solve it, but can change your perception of it, then do that. If you can't solve it or change your perception of an issue, then practice radical acceptance."[29]

We practice radical acceptance when we let go of judgement and see things as they really are. When we stop resisting reality and relax our body, we're in acceptance. It's radical when we examine our expectations to see if they are realistic, and focus on decisions that improve our well-being. Taking time to breathe deeply and checking our emotions will curb the temptation to participate in destructive behavior. We live in the present moment knowing we can only control our attitudes and actions – not anyone else's. It's radical when we love and have compassion for ourself, because often we're harder on ourself than others. Only then can we have love and compassion for other people. An open mind and patience will help us cultivate the courage, flexibility and resilience needed to navigate our way to radical acceptance.

When we can get beneath our emotions and connect with caring, both courage and clarity become available. This allows us to be present to ourself and others who may be experiencing a painful situation. Remembering our togetherness enhances our resilience. Loving ourself and using compassion to fuel our radical acceptance isn't always easy, but it is rewarding. It's radical acceptance that keeps us from becoming stuck in anger and bitterness, and rewards us with peace and serenity in difficult situations. We all need kindness when we're struggling, so let's begin with kindness to ourself as we step into radical acceptance of what we can't change.

RELEASING WHAT NO LONGER WORKS

Taking some time to think about what is
no longer serving us can be a life changer.
When we feel stressed, discontented, or
overwhelmed, we are experiencing indicators that something isn't

working. Some of the culprits that can keep us from moving into the life of contentment and peacefulness we want to live are possessions, habits, health, attitudes, relationships, or responsibilities.

A look into nature shows us that lizards and snakes shed their skins, and trees shed their bark because they have outgrown that skin or bark, and need to create new growth to continue a healthy life. We too need to shed what we have outgrown for our continued health. Clinging to the familiar is easier than letting go, but it stunts our growth to hold onto what is no longer appropriate for our job, stage of life, health, or current relationships.

When my husband and I moved full time to Florida, we chose a moderate size condo that was just right for the two of us. Our Michigan home would not fit into our condo, so like shedding a skin we donated books, games, clothing, and furniture. The goal was not to bring more than we needed. After arriving we discovered we still had too much which led to more donating, until we had what finally works for us now. We had to work through some of the emotional attachments we had to certain items collected over the years, but the lightness and freedom we felt in releasing things that no longer worked for this later stage of life was rewarding.

Physical baggage is easier to see and take care of than mental, emotional, or spiritual baggage. Mental, emotional, and spiritual baggage can remain in the background where unresolved issues slowly collect and build until, if there is no release, we reach a tipping point. Our body or mind may become unhealthy. Releasing what no longer works is a necessary step to achieving improved health, a calm mind, and balanced emotions.

Let's release playing the past over and over again wishing things were different. We don't need to be defined by our past, we can define our self by who we are now. Carl Jung wrote, "I am not what happened to me, I am what I choose to become."[30] The past no longer serves us, so let's release the fear that holds us back and embrace the present.

Let's release relationships that we thought were going to be different than they are. It could be a professional relationship with a medical doctor, or counselor that isn't working. Years ago, I was looking for a counselor and went through three before I found one that was the right fit. In our personal relationships our spouse, partner, or friends change and grow over time, as we do, and sometimes that means we outgrow a relationship that is stuck in unhealthy behavior.

Let's release grudges, anger, and resentment, and practice forgiveness. It's a waste of time and energy to think we can control anyone else, so let's concentrate on our own behavior. Hanging onto grudges, anger, and resentment is like being in jail with the key to get out and choosing not to use it. We can free ourselves by practicing forgiveness.

Let's release ourselves from what other people think of us, and instead make our priority what we think of our self. We can't live our values, and at the same time live concerned about what other people think about us. Mahatma Gandhi said, "Happiness is when what you think, what you say, and what you do is in harmony."[31] This quote reflects living our values, which is where life satisfaction comes from.

Let's release calling our self ugly names when we make mistakes, and release the fear of trying something new. Trying something new and making mistakes go together - it's how we learn to live life well. And how about lightening up and taking our self less seriously. Life feels so much better when we laugh, especially if we can laugh at our mistakes while we're learning from them.

Although something may have been valuable at one time, it's healthy to release it when it's no longer needed. This is not a process that is done quickly, it's a process that is repeated again and again over our lifetime as our bodies, relationships, and circumstances continue to change. We can regularly check in with ourselves to see if we're carrying any unnecessary baggage. Traveling with too much baggage means we trip and stumble over what we're trying to carry. It's time to free our self from what no longer works. Ask yourself if there isn't at least one thing you'd like to let go of and see if that doesn't make a difference.

RUNNING ON EMPTY

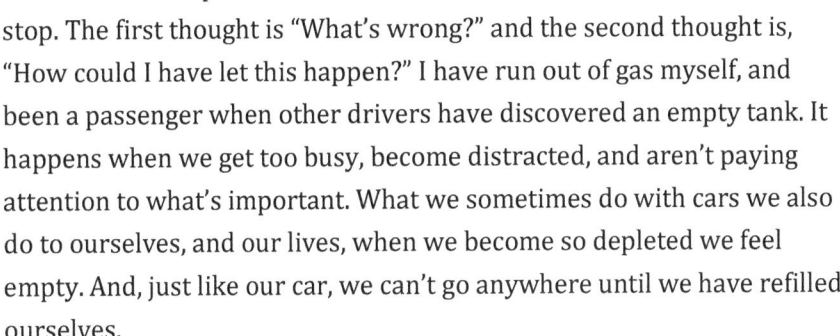

You know the awful feeling that happens when the car starts to sputter, and then rolls to a stop. The first thought is "What's wrong?" and the second thought is, "How could I have let this happen?" I have run out of gas myself, and been a passenger when other drivers have discovered an empty tank. It happens when we get too busy, become distracted, and aren't paying attention to what's important. What we sometimes do with cars we also do to ourselves, and our lives, when we become so depleted we feel empty. And, just like our car, we can't go anywhere until we have refilled ourselves.

Psychology expert Dr. Margaret Paul believes that inner emptiness is caused by a lack of self-love. "When we don't love ourselves, we look for approval from others, at the expense of our own needs and feelings. It's the peril we face when we listen to what others tell us about who we should be, and ignore who we really are. We waste our time and energy by filling our emptiness with distractions such as; work, food, shopping, unhealthy relationships, phone time, or TV binging. We don't run any better than a car does when the tank is empty."[32]

Ranata Suzuki writes, "Contrary to all logic and reason – emptiness hurts. You would not believe the pain and the suffering that can come from a thing which, by all accounts....is not even there."[33] But it is there, and, when we find our self in that empty place, we need to become aware of what is missing, what needs to be changed. We all have needs, but the painful part happens when our needs are not met.

If we're having trouble clarifying what we need, it can be helpful to talk to a trusted friend or respected counselor. Filling our empty selves begins with identifying what we value about our self and our life. That will help clarify priorities, so we can begin to refocus and rebalance. When we embrace our priorities, we begin to move from empty to filled. This allows us to live what author Trudi Griffin calls a "value-congruent" life, where our choices reflect our values.[34] This is living in fullness.

Emptiness can be a messenger telling us that we are starting to become more conscious. We're ready for change. It's one of those experiences that fit into being a blessing in disguise. As K. Hara writes, "Emptiness is the possibility yet to be filled."[35] A helpful place to start is with forgiveness for our imperfections. We're human and we're going to make mistakes. Let's give ourselves a break and practice mindfulness, which means being aware of our thoughts and feelings without judgement. We can experience the present moment, whatever it holds, without judgement. Judging ourselves empties us, but research shows mindfulness refills us because it can reduce stress and anxiety. This is a beautiful way to love our self.

Emptiness turns to "filled" when we practice healthy self-care seen in balancing sleep, diet, work, exercise, play, and relaxation into our daily lives. Even small improvements result in filling us up. Establishing a strong spiritual practice creates a peaceful mind that is focused on positive thinking. Spiritual practice is essential to what fulfills us, and makes our hearts sing. It is the source of love and deep inspiration.

We fill our empty places when we find beauty and meaning in everyday life. It's the small everyday things that put the larger context of our life into a positive perspective. Giving our full attention to whatever we're doing makes a big difference. This can be as simple as preparing a meal noticing all the colors, textures, and tastes involved, and turning it into a feast of appreciation. We fill ourselves when we keep our home environment pleasant and clutter free so we feel lifted when we enter our front door.

Appreciating what we have is another way to heal inner emptiness. Practicing gratitude centers our focus on what enhances our lives, creating positive energy. This means treasuring who we are right at this present moment. We can express our gratitude in our inner thoughts, journal writing, or out loud to those around us. Gratitude transforms whatever is happening and fills us to the brim.

When we feel we're running on empty, it's important not to become discouraged. Refueling takes time, and loving ourselves takes practice. It happens when we pursue what is important to us by taking small steps, one day at a time. What we go through always has a purpose, so let's pay attention to what life is trying to tell us. Let's keep each other encouraged as we all keep moving toward loving ourselves more fully. Life feels so much better when we stop running on empty and live out of fullness.

SACRED IDLENESS

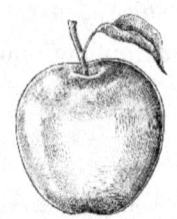

The skies were grey; the wind was steady;
and the rain constant throughout the day.
Project plans were set aside and the decision was made to nourish ourselves with a day of sacred idleness. For my husband and I that meant sharing thoughts uninterrupted, spending time with our current books, napping, eating leftovers so no cooking was needed, and letting our minds wander without any time constraints. It was wonderfully nurturing and left us ready to pick up our projects again with renewed energy and enthusiasm.

George Macdonald wrote, "Work is not always required of man. There is such a thing as sacred idleness, the cultivation of which is now fearfully neglected."[36] Both work and idleness can be sacred if kept in balance, which is a challenge in a society that overemphasizes action and busyness. Work activates mind and body while sacred idleness nourishes the soul, so both are needed – one is not more important than the other. But it is the sacred idleness that is most often neglected and we neglect it at our peril.

My husband, the pilot and engineer, reminded me of how important it is for an engine to idle. At a stop light a car rests, conserving its energy for moving forward when the light turns green. That time of rest conserves gasoline and wear on the engine, while increasing its productivity and life span. An airplane waiting to take off down the runway first goes through a complete engine check. Then it idles, conserving fuel, until cleared for takeoff. No engine can operate at full speed all the time without a breakdown in performance. What is true for machinery is also true for us – without idling we too break down.

The term sacred is often used in a religious setting, but it also includes anything that's highly valued, or set aside for a specific purpose. Sacred idleness is not about escaping reality, it's about making time for what renews our energy. It's about knowing what inspires us, what recharges our batteries. It's about pursuing small moments that matter like watching the waves while walking the beach, paying attention to the patterns of a camp fire, lounging in a chair feeling the sun on our skin, or spending time in our favorite garden spot, just looking and listening. It brings us into the present moment with relish.

For humans, the form sacred idleness takes is as varied as each one of us. For me this is especially current because I am in the middle of a major transition that requires careful decision making. To open myself to the wisdom of sacred idleness, I am doing something I have never done before. In February I am leaving town to intentionally go to a quiet retreat place without technology, schedules, or demands on my time. I will be silent during my stay and will make my own time line to hike, journal, ponder, nap, and embrace stillness, experiencing whatever arises. Out of this deep, sacred, idleness retreat will emerge the clarity, and discernment, needed for this transition. This is my time for the renewal and wisdom of sacred idleness.

Whatever your challenges are, dedicate some time to yourself. Embrace the gifts of sacred idleness and enjoy a renewed you.

SINGING OUR WAY TO BETTER HEALTH

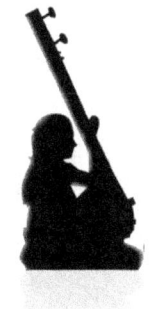

Instinctively we know that music and singing affect us. It's a language that crosses continents and cultures, and allows us to share uplifting experiences. Singing, by ourselves or in a group, not only lifts our spirits but also enhances our health. The best part is, a star quality voice isn't needed to have fun and reap the benefits. Decades of scientific evidence document that singing is good for our body, mind and spirit.

In the award-winning documentary film Alive Inside,[37] Dan Cohen, a social worker, went to a nursing home for people with dementia. Working with each person, he found out what music they liked and made a play list for them. As the residents listened to their personal choices, people who were barely talking proceeded to sing along to their music and dance. The outbreak of spontaneous singing took the staff by surprise. The door to their memory that had been closed for so long was now opening. The film concluded that both listening to music and singing reactivates the area of the brain that controls reasoning, speech, memory and emotion. So, singing improves cognition and clear thinking.

Researchers at a Harvard associated medical center have shown that singing helps people recover from strokes and brain injuries. Singing is part of the process to relearn speech. Former U.S. Representative Gabrielle Giffords[38] used song therapy to help her recover her ability to talk when a gun-shot wound to her head destroyed her speech. By singing first and then slowly dropping the melody, two years later she was able to testify before a Congressional committee. Even healthy people who sing learn words and phrases faster.

There are other benefits just waiting to be claimed with a song in the shower, or humming tunes on a road trip. Singing releases endorphins that make us feel good, and reduces the hormone cortisol so stress is reduced. The positive feelings of the endorphins can also help decrease pain. Singing can stimulate our immune system because it soothes us and lowers our blood pressure.

Patients in hospitals are able to calm themselves by singing their favorite songs. Their minds are quieted because fear and worry are reduced.

Recovering from surgery, my sister-in-law remembers one particular nurse that would walk the hall at night singing soothing songs. She remembers it because it was comforting to be sung to when she was in pain, and she could quietly hum along. Singing can be both a gift to ourself and others.

Singing improves lung function because it involves deep breathing and use of our respiratory muscles. This means that people who have asthma, cancer, COPD, and multiple sclerosis can benefit from singing. When we sing our posture is often improved. Regular singing can change breathing patterns enough to decrease snoring (my husband needs this one). This just keeps getting better and better.

Singing can help us process grief so it helps with emotional pain. I've sung to myself when I've needed a dose of serenity in the middle of something difficult. Songs don't have to be pretty - we can sing while we're crying which releases our pain, so healing can begin. Let's sing bravely when we're hurting and don't know what to do. Let's give voice to the anguish built up inside and let it out so a ray of hope, or peace, or relief can enter.

Whether it's singing or humming, it relaxes both body and mind, keeps us grounded and reduces unproductive thinking. Because it quiets the mind, we can more easily find our spiritual place of inner peace and serenity. What an amazing thing it is that our voice can carry healing energy throughout our body. Let's give ourself permission to break into song more often, or join a singing group for greater social connectedness. In Mitch Albom's words. "God sings, we hum along, and there are many melodies, but it's all one song – one same, wonderful human song."[39]

SOOTHING OURSELVES WHEN THE ROAD GETS ROUGH

No matter how skilled we are at managing life, there will be times when we experience unexpected events that make the road so rough, we lose our balance. During these times of sudden change or loss, using the skill of soothing ourself is essential to our mental health. Anything that produces a strong emotional reaction 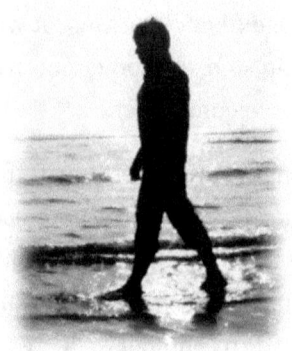 can be countered by comforting ourself. This lowers our stress so our mind stops racing, we breath more deeply and think with clarity.

I discovered I was better at soothing others than I was at comforting myself, so I expanded my skills and realized that this is not difficult to learn. It's a process of self-discovery that allows each of us to find what works. We gain a better understanding of ourself as we work on our emotions of loss, fear, sadness or anger.

Let's keep our self-soothing healthy and avoid binge eating, too much alcohol, an overdose of retail therapy or anything in excess. These are ways of avoiding difficult feelings which only makes them more powerful. Knowing how to sooth ourself helps us to process what's happening, so we can clarify our thoughts and manage our emotions in a way that reduces their power to unbalance us.

With that in mind let's explore some healthy options for comforting ourself. When I'm angry or upset, going for a walk – actually it's more of a stomp – helps me release my fear and negativity. Then I'm able to see what's most important to deal with first. Journaling is another way of working out strong emotions. We can give the paper a full description of how we are at this moment and it will be a release that won't hurt anybody else while it makes us feel better.

We can cook a favorite meal, walk the beach, watch the wind in the trees or the clouds changing shapes. There's snuggling with our pets or children, playing a musical instrument or listening to calming music. And, there's always the comfort of having a good cry which lowers our stress hormones and calms our heart rate.

Psychologist Dr. Julia Kogan[40] supports breathing deeply. Her research shows it produces a calming response by decreasing heart rate, blood pressure, and muscle tension as well as clearing our mind. We can enjoy the slow movement of a hammock or rocking chair, or curling up for a nap with a soft blanket and a mug of our favorite hot beverage. Then there's a long soak in a warm bath with a lit scented candle. That could be followed by a favorite lotion and a foot massage.

I think eating our favorite flavor chocolate belongs on the comfort list. I also enjoy the comforting quality of sitting by a window and listening to bird songs outside. We can phone someone we love and have a chat or meet them somewhere for coffee. Spending time with supportive people can be a powerful soother. Inspirational quotes and spiritual literature are comforting. There's prayer, guided meditation, yoga or tai chi. We can talk to ourself compassionately with kind and loving words that offer balance and perspective. The possibilities are endless and each of our comforting activities is shaped by our own needs.

No one escapes the strong feelings of unexpected events. Jonice Webb Ph.D. writes "Being able to tolerate and sooth a painful feeling makes you more resilient."[41] Learning to sooth ourself is essential. Let's discover what comforts us so we can manage a rough road with confidence, resilience and clarity.

THE ART OF MONO-TASKING

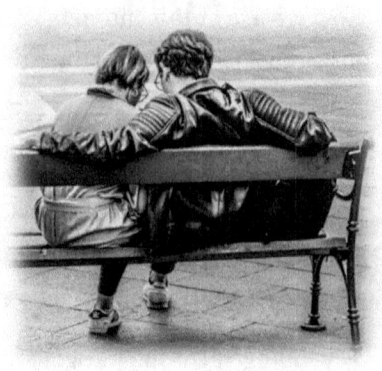

To appreciate the art of mono-tasking (doing one thing at a time) we first need to look at multi-tasking (doing several things at a time). When the temptation to do too much is high let's take an honest look at this and give ourselves a break. We live in a culture that wants us to juggle eight things at once, and get everything done yesterday. The message is that multitasking is the way to get there.

In our device laden world, we are encouraged to believe we can successfully navigate numerous tasks in a short period of time. Praise is offered to those who are the busiest. Feeling extremely productive can be so alluring that we buy into the myth of multi-tasking, and then experience its unintended consequences.

There is now new scientific evidence supporting the alarming consequences of multi-tasking. Our brains are not wired to rapidly switch from one task to another, so there is a cognitive cost. A recent study found the following. There was a reduction in the brains ability to regulate the brains control over both motivation and emotion. Our short-term and long-term memory is reduced, and we become easily distracted jumping between tasks.

Distractions cause us to misjudge traffic, experience more falls, perform lower in tasks, and have trouble making decisions. Our relentless juggling act increases chronic stress, depression and social anxiety. In the middle of life's daily activities, doing too much harms our valued relationships. Have you ever tried to have a conversation with someone who kept checking their phone and couldn't give you eye contact? This is what researchers are talking about when they say that lack of attention lowers relationship satisfaction. Now you can see why I said research results are alarming.

Researchers clearly found that rapidly switching tasks made people less productive and less efficient. This reveals the true results of multi-tasking. Being busy is not the same as being productive.

Let's reclaim the art of doing one thing at a time. Let's reclaim the pleasure of being mindful, and noticing the details of what we are doing. Let's reclaim the deep satisfaction of paying attention to our relationships with focused, nurturing behaviors. When we concentrate on one task, instead of several, we can give that one item our complete attention and our best effort. This often leads to greater enjoyment of what we're doing and can greatly improve the outcome.

Making a list of what's most important to us will help us create a focus. We can set times when we're digital free so we nurture ourselves, and then we can set times for getting together with supportive people. Done without interruption, both enhance our health and relationships. As Steve Jobs says, "Be like a postage stamp. Stick to one thing until you get there."[42]

When we are strategic with our time, we get everything done that truly needs to be done, without the constant stress to do more. All daily chores and errands become elevated and enjoyed when done thoughtfully. Mono-tasking offers us life's simple pleasures so we hear the different sections of the orchestra, smell the aroma from what's baking in the oven, feel the crispness of the clean sheets, or taste the robust flavor of a favorite drink.

Single tasking gives us the opportunity to notice when a neighbor looks distressed and needs a kind message of encouragement. We're aware of the sparkle in a child's eyes. We notice the sweetness of an elderly couple holding hands, slowed by their years, but still walking the beach. These are precious moments so easily missed.

I'm suggesting we exchange multi-tasking for mono-tasking. This means we exchange scattered minds for mindfulness, and rushing for thoughtful choices. Let's leave behind the temptation to know everything at once, and the fear that we'll miss out on something, to embrace the art of doing one thing at a time. It has been said the having at least one lazy day a week can reduce stress, high blood pressure, and the risk of having a stroke.[43] If that's all it takes, I'm in!

Let's make our celebrations focused on the people we love. This is an opportunity to carefully choose priorities, respect our tired brains, and meaningfully do less. Storm Jameson writes, "The only way to live is to accept each minute as an unrepeatable miracle, which is exactly what it is: a miracle and unrepeatable."[44] Welcome to the art of mono-tasking.

WHAT'S THE RUSH?

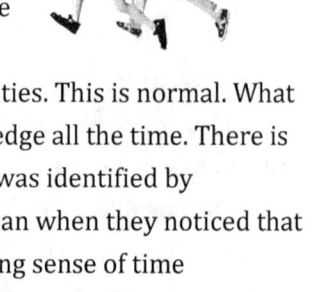

As we move through different stages of life, we all have times when we feel pressured and hurried to fulfill expectations and responsibilities. This is normal. What isn't healthy is finding ourself rushed and on edge all the time. There is an actual illness named "hurry sickness" that was identified by cardiologists Meyer Friedman and Ray Roseman when they noticed that many of their patients suffered from a "harrying sense of time urgency."[45] Hurrying steals our best. The faster we go, the more we miss out on what matters most. It leaves us feeling exhausted, empty, and stuck with the attention span of a gnat.

A few years ago, I found myself rushing across town clutching the steering wheel and elevating my blood pressure, so I could get to a yoga class on time. I didn't settle down until the end of class missing its full benefit. Then I ran a number of errands, raced to another appointment, and finished up with some grocery shopping before heading home where a project was waiting my attention. That evening I was exhausted and decided that it isn't the person with the most insane schedule that wins, it's the person who knows how to pace themselves and enjoy what they're doing that appreciates life the most.

Why do we do this to ourselves? It could be because we buy into our culture's affirmation of continuous accomplishments and the fear of appearing unproductive. There are also inner reasons why we do this. Kierkegaard once said, "The press of busyness is like a charm."[46] This means we feel important when our adrenaline is pumping. Thinking that constant activity may make us feel needed, liked, or admired, we choose to keep going. We may be chasing some moment of happiness available as soon as we get our to do list done.

If we feel like we are doing more than ever before, but not enjoying the rewards of our labor, we need to reevaluate. According to researchers, here are some of the signs of "hurry sickness." I identified with getting irritated with slow drivers in the left lane. Hurried people can't sit still and feel everything is urgent. They talk, think and walk fast, and are constantly worrying. They are exhausted but continue to multi-task, don't want to take breaks, and live by their watch. Eating is hurried and not enjoyed. Any of this sound familiar?

It's only when we slowdown that we realize what we're missing. I miss doing high quality work when I'm rushing because I'm prone to making more mistakes. The big picture gets lost in the stress of urgent details. Our ability to make sound decisions is affected because our brains are looking for quick answers, instead of the best solution. We miss down time which is critical to our wellbeing so we're exhausted. Peacefulness and contentment are gone. Most importantly, meaningful conversations and deep relationships are not built because texting at a stop light doesn't create that. We miss quality time with the people we love. Ann Voskamp writes, "In our rushing, bulls in a china shop, we break our own lives."[47]

How do we stay away from "hurry sickness"? At the top of the list is slowing down and taking the pressure off having to "get it done". We do this by choosing times to disconnect from our various devices, slowly eliminating commitments to anything unnecessary, opening our schedules, and practicing thoughtfulness. Then we can prioritize and connect with what truly matters. Let's realize love and concern for people is not necessarily compatible with hurrying. It's time to believe that we are not measured in what we do, but in who we are. Know that at the end of life, it is our ability to love and be loved that is our greatest legacy.

As Francis de Sales writes, "Never be in a hurry; do everything quietly and in a calm spirit. Do not lose your inner peace for anything whatsoever, even if your whole world seems upset. What is anything in life compared to peace of soul?"[48]

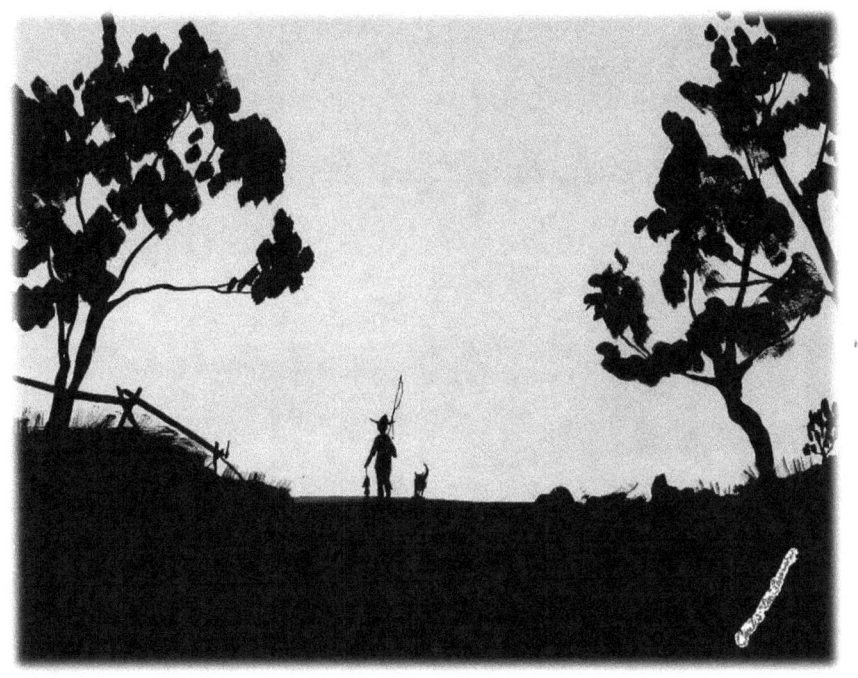

Chapter 5 - Life Skills

BECOMING SELF-AWARE

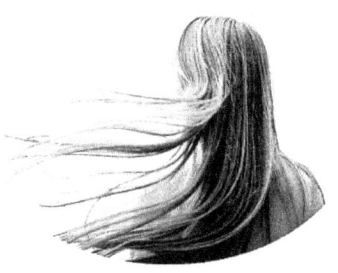

Recently, I took time away from family and responsibilities to cultivate deeper self- awareness in the face of unexpected events. This was needed for considering upcoming changes, and understanding what I needed in the process. The author Garima Srivastava writes, "Self-awareness is about understanding your own needs, desires, failings, habits, and everything else that makes you the unique individual you are. The more you know yourself, the better you are to adapting to life's changes."[1] I definitely needed to better understand myself and adapt to what life was giving me.

There are important advantages to living with heightened self-awareness. A better understanding of ourselves empowers us to build on our areas of strength, as well as clarify where we need to make improvements. This means paying attention to what is going on both inside and outside ourselves. When we're paying attention, we pursue opportunities that fit our skills and preferences. We better identify our stressors so we can more effectively use coping mechanisms. We understand our personal triggers, what we value most, the feelings involved, and the different roles we play in life. Our choices become consistent with our ability to make informed decisions, monitor our own behavior, and have healthy interactions with other people.

Change can take so many forms and challenge us in our deepest places. Those of us who have had a serious illness know all about the kind of change that turns our life upside down. The same is also true for caregivers. Here is where non-judgmental self-awareness is needed, and kindness to our self is essential. This is where we especially need to quiet the chatter in our minds, and switch off our "autopilot", so we can evolve into seeing the present moment clearly. It's in the self-awareness of the present moment that we have the power to positively change the way we see ourselves, and improve the quality of our life.

There are so many ways we can increase our self-awareness so only a few will be mentioned here. Try becoming more observant of your surroundings and sensations by noticing the breeze brushing past you, the scent of blooming jasmine, the soft soap in your hand, the flavor of your favorite food. Eat mindfully so every bite is enjoyed and you are aware of what you are putting inside yourself. Keep observing what you are thinking and feeling without judgement – just notice what is going on inside of you. Keep a journal where you write down thoughts and feelings about what you struggle with, and what you're grateful for. Read books about inspirational people. Practice listening to others which will enable you to listen with more compassion to yourself. Create a space for yourself where you can experience the gifts of meditation. Take a series of slow deep breaths. Spend time with people who are different from you so you can gain a new perspective and experience a fuller picture of yourself and others. All of these are life enhancers.

We may not be in control of the changes that continually present themselves, but we certainly can control how we handle them. The more self-aware we are, the more we can improve our quality of life. When we choose to be consciously in the present moment, awareness takes place and we develop skillful ways to handle the stress in our lives. May your self-awareness grow today.

CALLING ON COURAGE

Courage is needed for all our activities and
endeavors, even the most basic ones. Without it
we would be crippled by fear, and unable to meet
any of life's challenges. Courage is a choice, but
what does it look like? Here are a few examples. It
is a courageous act to leave our parent's home and
create an independent life of our own, and, if we
have overcome an abusive childhood, homelessness, or prejudice of any
kind, we have actually called on courage repeatedly. To love another
person and make a commitment to them, as in marriage, parenthood, or
long-lasting friendships, takes tremendous courage. Facing a serious
illness, career changes, and growing old all take courage.

It takes courage to work through our times of despair to a place of peace.
It's seen when we show our authentic self. Courage is part of choosing
our battles thoughtfully, instead of unconsciously reacting to a situation.
Courage shows when we choose perseverance over quitting, choose
responsibility over checking out, and progress over stagnation. Courage
sets boundaries for healthy relationships. And when we choose love over
fear and creation over destruction, we are again calling on courage.
Brené Brown writes in her book Rising Strong, "I believe that what we
regret most are our failures of courage, whether it's the courage to be
kinder, to show up, to say how we feel, to set boundaries, to be good to
ourselves."[2]

To me courage is showing up for life with a willingness to step into
change, discomfort or uncertainty with an open heart. It's about being
real when maintaining the status quo would be much easier. It's about
living personal priorities, not just talking about them. Courage
acknowledges fear, but chooses to take the next needed step. In John

Wayne's words, "Courage is being scared to death.... and saddling up anyway."[3] I've been a volunteer in an equestrian therapy program and seen several women, visibly afraid of the horse, get into the saddle and ride despite their fear. Because courage is contagious, other women were inspired to give riding a try and not one of them regretted working through their fear. In fact, they enjoyed heightened self-confidence and were eager to try more new activities.

Our individual journeys will challenge us in ways we can't even imagine, so where can we find the courage to meet those challenges? On a spiritual level courage comes from deep within. When we turn to our Higher Power (God, Universe, Great Spirit, whatever name works for you), we are given access to guidance that clarifies our perspective, intention, and decision making. We are supported with higher wisdom.

Courage comes from the support of people who believe in us. Their faith in us creates confidence because, if they believe in us, it is easier for us to believe in ourselves. As they share their time, resources, and words, we gain new perspective for the challenge we face. Encouragement from people we trust helps us manage negative thoughts and fears. Albert Schweitzer writes, "In everyone's life, at some time, our inner fire goes out. It is then burst into flame by an encounter with another human being. We should all be thankful for those people who rekindle the inner spirit."[4]

Our own intuition is a source of courage. Those inner nudges about needed changes are important messages meant for guidance. It's also another way our Higher Power communicates. Intuition can tell us to change our driving route, and later we discover there was a major accident on the route you were originally considering. Intuition tells us to leave a dangerous situation, go to a different doctor, or change jobs. Any change takes courage, and the more we listen to our intuition, the easier it will be to call on courage.

Experience is another source of courage. When we look at past experiences, and the resources that came our way just when they were needed, we build confidence in our ability to call on courage again. Our struggles reveal our character because it is in our darkest moments that we find out who we really are. Calling on courage gives us the power to meet our challenges with strength, no matter how frightening life may look. Ralph Marston writes, "Every fear is an opportunity to grow in confidence and courage. Face the fear, and find the power of your courage."[5]

We're all in the process of becoming who we came to the planet to be. Our problems don't need to hold us hostage. Let's call on the power of courage, and have faith in the growth process of our journey. Let's trust the people we are becoming, and call on courage together.

EMBRACING CHANGE AND FINDING "ISLANDS OF STABILITY"

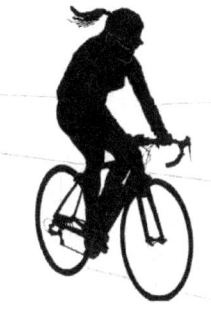

The last two months have given new meaning to the idea of living with change. Change is always a constant, but its recent accelerated rate has presented more than the usual challenge. When change is painful, we often act with resistance, which creates another set of problems that can manifest as frustration, anger, or depression. The status quo is often preferred. In order to embrace change we first need to acknowledge it.

Then, difficult as it is, we need to accept change. That means looking realistically at what we can and can't change. We can't control other people's motives, attitudes, shopping habits, broken promises or addictions. What we can control is our own attitude. We can choose to create fun at home, limit news and social media, and act with kindness and compassion. Practicing quiet mindfulness and meditation will move us from stress and anxiety, to accepting impermanence, and even embracing it.

If we're going to embrace change, we need to start with our self. Marianne Williamson, in her book **The Gift of Change** writes, "The most important factor in determining what will happen in our world is what you decide to let happen within you. Every circumstance — no matter how painful — is a gauntlet thrown down by the universe, challenging us to become who we are capable of being. Our task, for our own sakes and the sake of the world, is to do so."[6] When we are in the middle of painful circumstances, it isn't what happens to us, it's what we do with it that will make the difference.

In his book **In Future Shock**[7], Alvin Toffler refers to what he calls "islands of stability." He says these are especially needed when change is rapid, and it refers to the elements in our lives that don't change. These become our anchors. What are your "islands of stability?" A few of mine are my Higher Power, my spouse, treasured longtime friends, and feeling connected with my community. It's staying in touch with family (either biological or chosen), reading inspiring literature, and going outside biking or walking with the wind in my hair and the sun on my face. Another "island of stability" is quiet meditation. I'm sure you can add to the list.

When we relax into change, and embrace it, we recognize we are growing stronger, even when we're afraid. We learn we aren't easily broken, and move into a realm of calmness, peace, and courage. And from that emerges our growing wisdom. It is the reward for the hard work of navigating the storm because it strengthens the anchor that keeps us balanced and centered. It helps us establish a much needed new normal.

Embracing change ushers in an opportunity to support, love, share resources, respect, encourage, promote equality, and practice kindness.

In Brené Brown's words, "We are being given an opportunity to stitch a new garment. One that fits all of humanity and nature."[8] it isn't often we have a chance to make changes of this significance. Let's fully embrace any challenge by acknowledging it, accepting what we can and can't control, finding our "islands of stability," and pursuing the wisdom that is the reward for working through any change. The learning curve can be steep but we have our growing selves, and each other, and both are a treasure! Let's summon our most courageous selves to embrace, and even welcome change, knowing that we will be kinder, stronger, and wiser because of the experience. Let's meet each other in a place of calmness and peace. No one is in this alone — isn't that a comfort!

FINDING HOPE

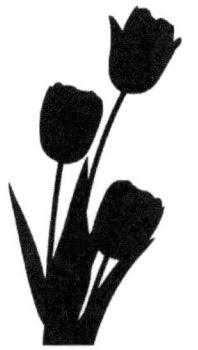

Yesterday, after calling my doctor with flu like symptoms, I was given an appointment time, and told to go to the drive through Convid-19 testing center outside Cleveland Clinic Indian River Hospital. Following instructions, I sat in the left side back seat while my husband drove. We were greeted by a police officer who verified my appointment with waiting medical staff, then we followed the cone marked drive to the testing site. The test itself is unpleasant, but quick and painless. We will have results in 4 – 7 days.

On the way home we talked about our strategy for doing what we can to protect Curt, who is currently healthy. Our living space is now divided in half so Curt is at one end, and I am at the other. It's separate togetherness. We each have a bed and a bathroom, and Curt is now "King of the Kitchen," which he enjoys. It had been 12 days since I had been out to pick up groceries, and a prescription; I am wearing a mask and gloves. Now we're home full time. Our groceries are being delivered.

 I have read numerous heart wrenching Convid-19 stories, featuring the difficult decisions doctors must make concerning who gets to use lifesaving equipment. In the middle of this situation the word hope came to mind. We need hope no matter what form a crisis takes. I'm anticipating I have no more than the average flu, but if that's not the case, where do I to find hope?

Hope is cultivated with faith in a Higher Power. There is so much out of our control that knowing that there is a Higher Power and it abides within me is comforting, and gives me hope. Keeping ourselves spiritually healthy helps us stay positive, when it is so easy to drown in negative news reports; in this case a pandemic. If we remove our focus from what we can't control, to what is in our control, we improve our mental, spiritual, and physical health. The biggest thing we can control is our attitude. Virginia Satir writes, "Life is not the way it's supposed to be, it's the way it is. The way you cope is what makes the difference."[9] For me, combining my faith in a Higher Power, and following all the protective health guidelines I am being given right now, fosters hope, and hopeful outcomes. Whatever happens, I will embrace it knowing that this is happening for me, not to me.

Hope is found in gratitude. When we take time to look at all the loving relationships, meaningful work, shelter, food, and that package of toilet paper a neighbor sent, we build hope. When we acknowledge the beauty outside our windows, a thriving indoor plant, or the pleasure of comfort food, we lift our spirits. This is the time for a gratitude journal so we can identify at least three things we are thankful for every day. If that's too many just write one gratitude. When we show appreciation for the kindnesses that are a part of each day, even if we must look hard to find them, hope thrives. When more shows up to be grateful for, an even larger reservoir of hope is created.

Hope is found in learning from past difficult times. John Maxwell writes, "Facing difficulties is inevitable, learning from them is optional."[10] If we can incorporate lessons learned from the past, into hope for our present challenge, we strengthen our ability to meet a crisis with courage and compassion. Mistakes can be some of our best teachers because they clarify what we will do different the next time we problem solve. Past learned wisdom is an available and valued resource for building hope.

Hope is found in kindness, and that starts with being kind with ourselves. Sometimes we forget to give ourselves credit for what we have done well. This isn't being conceited – this is being honest in our recognition of accomplishments large and small. It also means we go to bed early when we're tired, say no to activities we know are not right for us, cry when we need to cry, and ask for help when we're overwhelmed. Kindness to others is a spirit booster, too. If we can't be together physically, we can reach out with a letter, phone text message, computer email, or use other social media. We can make a phone call, do Facetime, or Zoom®. Sometimes it's the little kindnesses that mean the most but, whether large or small, they always enhance hope.

So, while I wait for my test results, I will continue to have faith in my Higher Power, practice gratitude, remember lessons learned, and be kind to myself and others (especially my husband who is taking care of me right now!). Hope really isn't hard to find – it's everywhere if we are willing to look.

KEEP IT SIMPLE *Simplfy! Simplfy.—*

"Simplify, Simplify" is Henry David Thoreau's famous message from his retreat on Walden Pond. This the perfect time to look around to see what might need attention. If it's our sanity coming into question then it's definitely time for action.

The last thing we want to do is turn simplifying our lives into another impossible goal to meet. This doesn't need to be stressful. The key is to clarify our priorities. Once that is clear, it is a painless process to discard what no longer supports your life. It doesn't matter if it is clutter in closets, or a calendar full of commitments. By simplifying we will relieve ourselves from the problems of having too much stuff or making more promises than can be kept.

My husband and I had the adventure of living in England for 3 years. The little house we rented offered us 800 square feet of living space. That was considerably smaller than our American home. Much to our surprise, we were perfectly content in that small space, and grateful we did not have more to take care of. That was the beginning of a major life style change for us. Since then, we have continued to downsize in every area of our lives.

The reward is a feeling of lightness (like we have just lost 100 pounds) that comes from being unencumbered by anything that doesn't fit who we are now. Time that was spent taking care of things is now spent taking healthier care of ourselves. Letting go of what is no longer needed frees us to embrace more personal time, couple time, friend time and community service. Our purchasing rule now is – if we bring something new into our home, then something similar that we already have is donated to a community organization that reuses things like Goodwill or Habitat for Humanity.

Peter Walsh, a professional home organizer, says that our homes are an outer reflection of our inner life (hard to believe, but true). First we better check on our inner life. So, clearing emotional clutter out of our "mind closet" is a good place to begin simplifying. Order within then begins to materialize in the order of our outer home.

We can continue to simplify by eliminating one stressful item from the calendar, going through one shelf or drawer, stepping out of Facebook for a while, or streamlining self-care so we feel good without being exhausted. Other changes that help simplify are; slow down, do one thing at a time, resist interruptions, take time off, shorten phone calls, put people first, and practice polite refusals to people requesting more time and energy than we have to give.

Let's support and encourage each other to let go of what no longer serves us well, and embrace the simplicity that is vital to our health and wellbeing.

LIFE'S LITTLE PLEASURES

My husband held out the phone to me saying, "It's a hospital nurse calling." We had been waiting for the results of my Convid-19 test. I felt my heart rate increase as I held the phone and listened. Several days earlier we had been told by another nurse, that if one person in the home has coronavirus, they assume everyone will get it, so no one else in the house will be tested. My husband's lungs are not as strong as mine, so I had been concerned.

Hearing the nurse say that there was no Convid-19 evidence in my test produced a huge sigh of relief. She laughed when I said, "I have never been so glad to have good old plain, ordinary, flu!"

A few days were still needed for my full recovery, but I was already starting to feel better. During my time of illness, I experienced a heightened awareness of life's little pleasures. Some came from Curt who made sure I always had a glass of something to drink close by, filled our home with delicious smells from the kitchen, and gave me numerous encouraging messages. When kitchen supplies ran low there was the pleasure of hearing the doorbell ring, announcing the arrival of fresh groceries. Texts (they don't have to be long to be meaningful) from loved ones lifted my spirits, along with loving advice from our granddaughter (a nurse who is working in a Convid-19 wing of a hospital).

Why wait to be sick to appreciate small enjoyments. Now that I'm back on my feet, I want to continue to be aware of life's little pleasures. They fill all of our days, if we're willing to look. Edward M Hays writes, "When we lack proper time for the simple pleasures of life, for the enjoyment of eating, drinking, playing, creating, visiting friends, and watching children at play, then we have missed the purpose of life. Not on bread alone do we live but on all these human and heart-hungry luxuries."[11]

We are the curators of our own contentment, so relishing these simple moments is a daily present to our self. Many of these small pleasures don't cost anything, or are inexpensive, so they're available to all of us. And the happiness they bring deepens our awareness of how many of these gifts each day offers. Now is a perfect time to identify and share these delightful experiences with each other. Here are a few of mine.

≪The smell of soup simmering on the stove

≪Hearing the front door close and knowing Curt is home

≪Settling into the recliner with my current book

≪Taking that first bite of a totally decadent dessert

≪Listening to mourning doves outside my window

≪Walking a nature trail

≪A long hot bath with lots of bubbles

≪Fresh sheets on my bed

≪Blowing bubbles with young children

≪TV movie night with popcorn

≪Laughing at embarrassing moments

≪Eating by candlelight

≪Wrapping up in my favorite soft blanket

≪A cat settling into my lap and purring

≪An unexpected compliment

≪Holding hands with someone I love

≪Listening to music

≪Watching a colorful sunset

≪Visiting the library

≪Visiting friends

Many more could be mentioned. These events add depth and delight to the day, no matter what is happening in life. We can take this opportunity to notice, and share, the simple things that add pleasure to our days. What small things bring you happiness? Does anyone like to pop bubble wrap besides me? As Paulo Coelho says, "It's the simple things in life that are the most extraordinary."[12]

MAKING SOMEDAY TODAY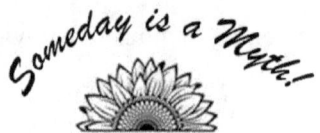

We have all heard people say they are going to take a trip, mend a relationship, finish a project, or take care of themself someday, as though someday was guaranteed. A colleague of my husband saved all his travel plans for when he retired, only to pass on less than a year after retiring. He never had his someday. Rachel Hollis writes, "Stop waiting for someday; someday is a myth. Don't wait to have the time; start planning to make the time."[13] We can choose to make someday today.

Often the culprit is procrastination. In an article, Elizabeth Lombardo Ph.D.[14] writes that procrastination leads to increased stress, health problems, poor performance, sleep issues, and regret. It also hinders self-esteem because self-critical thoughts result from putting off tasks and goals.

Perfectionism is one of the biggest reasons for procrastination. If we wait until everything is perfect, we fall into an all-or-nothing mentality which is certainly counter-productive. This holds us back from starting or completing anything. Have you ever heard of anyone procrastinating their way to success? Let's relieve ourself from the burden of being perfect and make someday happen today.

Sometimes we put relationships that need mending on our someday list. This is especially hard if there has been a betrayal of trust, or a major difference in politics or religion. We may tell ourself that we'll forgive that person after they apologize and make amends. However, that person will be just fine whether we forgive them or not. The person we're hurting is ourself with our harbored anger and bitterness. Remember, bitterness is like drinking poison and expecting the other person to die.

Let's remember that we don't need to agree on everything to maintain a friendship, but we do need to be clear on our non-negotiables and set boundaries. If the friendship needs to end, we can forgive and let go. If the relationship damage is minor, we can make a date to meet, talk through what happened with patience and empathy, and reestablish the communication and intimacy we previously enjoyed. Why put that off if the person is important to us?

If a trip is on our someday list, we can start by getting needed details, creating a trip fund, and finding a workable calendar date. Setting the goal is exciting, as is the pleasure of anticipation. It can be a trip across town, or to another continent, as long as it brings pleasure. A shorter trip to a beach, museum, library, or park can boost our spirits and make a day feel special. Life is meant to be enjoyed, not put on hold.

Are there any projects around the house on our someday list? If we're having trouble getting started, we can remind ourself of how good we'll feel once it's completed. Home projects can be either short or long-term activities. Things like organizing the basement, decluttering a closet, or cleaning the refrigerator, can be broken down into small daily increments that produce the satisfaction of completion in a few days. Then we can reward ourself for a job well done.

Taking care of ourself needs to be taken off our someday list and put on our today list. When it comes to our health, it's important to acknowledge that nagging problem and see a doctor. The cost of not doing that is too high. I've heard too many people say, "I wish I'd gone to the doctor sooner," or "I didn't know people my age could get cancer." Taking care of ourself also means nurturing our soul. This happens when we make quiet time to listen to our inner guidance. Our soul is also nourished when we embrace gratitude, practice kindness, laugh often, and love deeply.

Stephanie Klein writes, "Here's what I've learned about "soon"; it's short for "someday.""[15] "We make space in our lives for what matters, now. Not in promises and soon, but on mantels with sterling frames, in shelves we clear to make room for our now." Every day is a precious gift, so let's not put off doing what is most important. Let's make sure our choices are worthy of this one marvelous life, and take someday off hold. Someday can be today.

MAKING THE MOST OF OUR THRESHOLDS

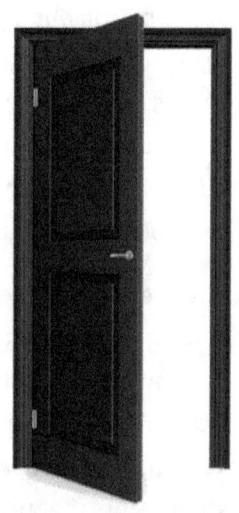

Standing at a threshold, which is a place of change, is a theme that repeats itself throughout our life. Thresholds can represent both large and small events, carrying a variety of emotions. It requires courage to step past the unsettledness of unanswered questions and venture into the unknown. It's easier to stay in the familiar and comfortable than risk the discomfort of not knowing what comes next. Thresholds invite us to review our choices, and discover new opportunities. They are game-changers that offer an invitation to become increasingly true to ourself.

Here is how John O'Donohue expresses this, "The word threshold was related to the word thresh, which was the separation of the grain from the husk or straw when oats were flailed. It also includes the notions of entrance, crossing, border, and beginning. To cross a threshold is to leave behind the husk and arrive at the grain."[16] This is a call for us to welcome our own inner richness.

Sometimes we can find ourself crossing a threshold we had never anticipated that feels like a sudden unchosen fork in the road. COVID certainly did that to all of us. We can ask ourself, what are we going to do with that threshold? How will we live differently after this experience? Kristin Armstrong writes, "Times of transition are strenuous, but I love them. They are an opportunity to purge, rethink priorities, and be intentional about new habits. We can make our new normal any way we want."[17] Thresholds are an invitation to change what needs changing.

Thresholds happen when we lose our job, an accident brings grief or we receive a health diagnosis we never expected to have. If we're considering a treatment plan or surgery, let's not let anyone push us into a decision we aren't ready to make. Thresholds can help us find our voice so we speak up in new ways.

There are also thresholds of celebration such as weddings, a baby's arrival, birthdays, job promotions, graduations and retirements. The beginning of each day is a threshold – what will we do with this precious gift? When we connect who we are with how we live, there are shifts inside us that change our perspective. Our resistance to change decreases and we step more fully into our life.

Marilyn Tan wrote an article giving some helpful suggestions in navigating the transition of thresholds.[18] These can involve major life changes as well as subtle shifts in consciousness. She suggests we acknowledge something is ending instead of pretending nothing is changing. This helps us prepare for whatever is emerging. If we honor the transition, we can allow ourself to feel the emotions of uneasiness, sorrow, or delight as we give ourself time to process. There are always new insights into ourself and others when something is either ending or beginning. Seeking support is essential whether we're celebrating or commiserating, and this strengthens our connections. When we let go of our fear and self-limiting beliefs, we can exercise the power of choice and embrace the new opportunities thresholds offer.

Giving complete attention to our guiding inner voice enables us to trust the process we're in. John O'Donohue's describes thresholds as, "voyages of discovery, creativity and compassion." He also adds, "No threshold need be a threat, but rather an invitation and a promise. Whatever comes, the great sacrament of life will remain faithful to us, blessing us always with visible signs of invisible grace. We merely need to trust."[19]

MAKING THE WRONG TURN AND FINDING THE RIGHT WAY

My husband and I were deeply engaged in conversation while driving to Orlando Sanford International Airport to pick up our

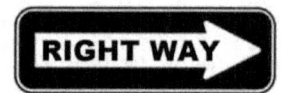

son and grandson. We were looking forward to greeting them with hugs at the airport when they came down the escalator. This trip to the airport had been made numerous times in the past, but this time we were too busy talking and missed our normal exit. The next exit, 12 miles further, put us in completely new territory. We wondered where we were and if we would get to the airport in time to greet them.

Scrambling for new route directions, we discovered another road that was a direct connection to the airport. When we arrived at the airport and realized their flight had been delayed, we were gratefully able to watch them come down the escalator and give them an enthusiastic welcome. Our missed exit sent us in the wrong direction, but exploring new territory introduced us to another helpful route, and we arrived just where we were supposed to be and on time to meet them.

Here are two more examples. I've chosen both doctors and councilors that weren't right for me, and in choosing another found just what I needed. In the past I have been hard on myself when I didn't meet my own unrealistic expectations. After getting tired of feeling inadequate, I realized that when I accepted and loved myself just the way I was, I felt so good that my quality of work went far beyond what I was achieving when I was harshly judging myself. A poor decision turned into an important lesson and a much better way of living.

Sometimes what feels like a wrong choice can bring us to the right place, and what we learn along the way can be invaluable. We may discover we need to change cities, jobs, relationships, churches, attitudes, diet or exercise routines. If we're open, we'll see where we're not listening to life and our blind spots become evident.

Some people choose to make harmful decisions repeatedly like the man with very little money who spent $22,000.00 buying lottery tickets. When he died, he left his wife with very little. He never learned to responsibly handle money, but his children, watching their dad, made sure they did not follow his behavior. He was an example of continuous irresponsibility, but his children were not. Anyone with substance abuse issues is repeating the same mistakes, however, those who come out of that scenario to find themselves, and create a new life, have found the right way out of a wrong turn.

In an article, Carina Wolff[20] suggests some signs that indicate it's time to question the path we're on. When we do things for other people but not ourself, when our accomplishments aren't satisfying, when we question everything and feel uninspired, we need to reconsider our path. If we need to justify what we're doing and become defensive, we're lacking clarity about where we are and need to rethink our direction. Another clue is a feeling of anxiety that takes away our peace and serenity. When we continually question what we're doing we need to change direction. Any of this sound familiar?

Life does not need to be perfect to be enjoyed. Sometimes the decisions we make that feel like wrong turns take us to the very best outcomes. We recognize changing circumstances, see what works and what doesn't, and identify what matters most. Compassion is learned as well as forgiveness for ourself and others. We address the injustices in our life, reveal our true feelings, and know when it is time to move on. Wrong turns make us more authentic. They slow us down and remind us of the importance of pacing ourself. Our wrong turns are the basis for making different choices. We're only a decision away from the change we need to make.

It makes me wonder if turns are really wrong when they reveal insights, opportunities, lessons and positive changes. As my husband Curt says, "It isn't what you've done, it's who you've become." Let's take whatever we've done that felt like a mistake and transform our thinking, so, we can become a deeper, more compassionate person. Whatever detour may happen, when we've arrived with being comfortable, confident, and peaceful with the direction we're headed, our journey will be so much more rewarding and enjoyable.

"MIND THE GAP"

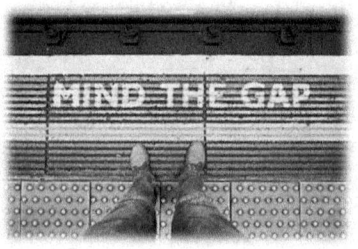

The London Underground rapid transit system first opened in 1863, making it the oldest rapid transit system in the world. Because of the space between the platform and the train, a recorded voice was installed in 1968 to warn travelers to "mind the gap" every time the train stops at a station. It has since become a brand name for everything from T-shirts, to door mats, to video games. These three words ask passengers to pay attention to the step between where they are and where they want to go.

Falling in the space between the platform and the train could cause serious injury.

I'd like to suggest that "mind the gap" is a prudent reminder to be thoughtful of this space in our life journey, represented by where we stand now, and where we want to go. We need to mind the gaps in our growth. When we're mindful, we increase our ability to choose wisely. Mindfulness can heighten our awareness of what is going on both inside and outside of ourselves, so we process what we see and feel before choosing to respond. This helps eliminate a thoughtless knee jerk reaction which would be equivalent to falling through the space between the platform and the train. Choosing if, when, and how to respond is a sign of personal growth, and illustrates a healthy "minding the gap."

When we have any serious illness, we "mind the gap" between where we are in our diagnosis, and where we want to be through treatment. After looking at our options, we choose what is best for us knowing that if changes are needed along the way we will make them.

In the middle of any major event, it's easy to get swept up in anxiety and fear, projecting the worst-case scenarios for the future. Viktor Frankl writes in his book **Man's Search for Meaning**, "Between stimulus and response, there is a space. In that space is our power to choose our response. In our response lies our growth and our freedom."[21] That space is where we "mind the gap." This is the time to make friends with uncertainty, no matter how uncomfortable that feels. Answers to managing a challenge may come slowly. We can choose to make thoughtful decisions, knowing we're doing our best, or we can react with anger and risk taking. This "gap" is too critical to fall through.

"Minding the gap" in relationships is also helpful. When relationships fall into predictable patterns, blind spots can develop and do serious damage. When we explore where we are and where we want to be in our relationships, we can identify what is working well and what needs to change. We take responsibility for our words and actions, and problem solve with honesty, vulnerability, and compassion. Each person's feelings are honored. Respect and shared values are as important as love in bridging the gap between a stagnant friendship, and a dynamic, growing bond. If a person becomes toxic, that is the time to end the connection because that "gap" can be destructive.

When it comes to taking on a new challenge there is the "gap" between what we want to do, and fear of failure. This is where we want to avoid letting yesterday's mistakes create fear for trying something new today. We "mind the gap" well when we treat past experiences as a helpful resource for future decisions, instead of a reason to avoid trying anything new. Henry Ward Beecher wrote, "We should not judge people by their peak of excellence; but by the distance they have travelled from the point they started."[22] Just trying something new is an accomplishment, no matter how it turns out.

My husband and I loved traveling through England and frequently used the Underground transit system. The phrase "mind the gap" brings back delightful memories and is a reminder to remember that there are many ways to get from where we are to where we want to be. Let's all enjoy the pleasure and success of looking at our lives and seeing clearly how we're helping ourselves get to where we really want to go. Let's "mind the gap" and remember to enjoy the journey!

NEED A REBOOT?

FRESH START

**PUSH TO
ACTIVATE**

All of us go through changes. Some are predictable like changing jobs, aging or parenthood. Others come as unexpected events such as the car breaking down, or a health crisis. When change happens, we may find ourself wondering how to handle our new circumstances. This is when we need to step back and, instead of letting fear take over, give ourself a reboot. This is not comparing people to computers, but using the term to indicate the desire to make a fresh start. New beginnings are the doorway to fresh perspective, creativity, and trust in our Higher Power.

How do we know when it's time for a reboot? Valerie Soleil[23] has researched signs that indicate it's time for a new beginning. She says that if we're feeling sad, miserable and unhappy, and what used to be enjoyable no longer brings us pleasure, we need a fresh start. Becoming angry and sinical means we need to give our mental health a reboot. When our body is changing and we feel continually tired, run down, have aches and pains that interfere with our usual routines and can't sleep, we need a change. If we're irritated easily and are quickly loosing our temper, we need a reboot. Finding ourself stuck in the past or future indicates we've lost the present moment, and need to restart our thought process.

Every day is a new beginning, so we can start over any time we choose. Let's start our reboot with patience, which means treating ourself with gentleness, love and compassion. Starting over requires courage, resilience, faith and an understanding of how limitations affect the quality of our life. This is where perspective comes in, because this is where we can change limitations into opportunities.

It's the way we look at our life that can make all the difference. All our experiences are derived from our perception of what is happening. Leon Ho writes, "Being able to control how you look at things is the key to learning how to start over. Shaping your perception is so powerful that just a small change in perspective can completely change everything, from your motivation and outlook, to your self-esteem and confidence."[24]

Our priorities may change over time, so part of a new beginning is identifying what is most important now. When that is clear we know where to invest our time and energy. Since life is ever changing, we need to embrace change and accept the situation as though we have chosen it. This can be difficult, but it is acceptance that can work miracles. We reboot when we breathe deeply and immerse ourself in the present moment.

Talking things over with our Higher Power can be a meaningful part of a new beginning, as is expressing gratitude for the precious gifts that are part of our life. Sometimes starting over means letting go of limiting beliefs, easy excuses and expectations about how life should be. Let's remember we are in a continuous process of becoming, and that process is helped when we listen to and trust our inner wisdom.

When we reboot, we can take baby steps, but baby steps are still effective. The result is increased happiness, new skills, empathy, confidence and a deeper sense of peace. We don't need to wait for big events to create the need for a reboot, we can choose to make everyday a new beginning. Luminita D. Saviuc writes, "Each day is a gift given by life itself. Each day is a new beginning, a new chance and a new opportunity for you to create something better, something new. To offer more value to the world around you, and to reveal more of yourself to those you love. Each day is a new life, each moment is a precious gift. So, let's make the best of each day and the most of each moment."[25]

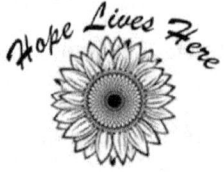

NO MATTER WHAT HAPPENS, THERE'S ALWAYS HOPE

Eva Kor is a holocaust survivor.[26] When she was 10, she and her twin sister were used in medical experiments by a doctor in Auschwitz. Eva was injected with a deadly germ and when the doctor saw how sick she was he laughingly said, "Too bad, she's so young – she has only two weeks to live." Eva knew she was very sick, but she made a vow to herself that she would survive, prove the doctor wrong, and be reunited with her sister Miriam.

Auschwitz certainly seems like a hopeless place but, during the next five weeks, as Eva faded in and out of consciousness, she reminded herself that she was going to get well, and see her sister. All she could control was crawling to a source of water and crawling back to bed again. But, she never stopped hoping. Slowly she improved, and finally she was released to return to her barracks, and her sister Miriam. Deep inside she knew that if she could survive that, she could survive anything. That experience gave her confidence in her ability to overcome difficulties, and she continues to use that skill to be ready for whatever the next life challenge might be.

In her adult life she became a forgiveness advocate and shared her story with many people. When people began to give Eva feedback on how her story helped them, she realized the power of hope filled stories. When we share how we've overcome our cancer, divorce, financial debt, job loss, depression, or passing of a loved one, others begin to believe they can too. This is hope in action. As Virginia Satir writes, "Life is not the way it's supposed to be, it's the way it is. The way you cope is what makes the difference."[27]

Just like Eva, we build hope when we focus on what we can control by putting all of our attention on what is in our power to change. We build hope when we stay positive. That doesn't mean we don't get discouraged or shed a few tears, it means we move forward by picking up the pieces and making needed changes. Gaining perspective from a difficult time means our actions are affected, so we don't stay in a hard place any longer than necessary.

Hope comes from taking any opportunity there is to actively improve our situation. For perspective we may need to step back and look at the big picture, so we notice all the details of our challenge, and clearly see our options. Barack Obama offers this advice, "The best way to not feel hopeless is to get up and do something. Don't' wait for good things to happen to you. If you go out and make some good things happen, you will fill the world with hope, you will fill yourself with hope."[28]

Hope takes time to see what there is to be grateful for at the end of each day. This is a good time to acknowledge how far we've come, and give ourselves credit for doing the best we know how to do. When we're kind to our self we're practicing hope. It's gentle self-care that helps us survive tough times, so let's engage our bodies and minds in meaningful nurturing.

Hope finds a light no matter how dark it is, and sometimes that light comes from our community. Surrounding ourselves with people who are loving, honest, and supportive, makes any difficult situation bearable. Steve Goodier sums this up well when he writes, "Who do you spend time with? Criticizers or encouragers? Surround yourself with those who believe in you. Your life is too important for anything less."[29]

Whatever the source or form of our tough time, it is essential to our wellbeing to practice forgiveness. This is what made the difference for Eva, and this is the foundation of hope. Our first reaction to any tough event may be anger and blame, but staying there will make the situation worse. To move forward, we need to stop obsessive thinking about the situation, release our judgements, and forgive whoever is involved. Sometimes that person is our self. If the problem we're facing is the direct result of something we've done, it's easy to become destructively self-critical. Self-forgiveness is just as essential as forgiveness of anyone else!

Eva Kor is a dramatic example of someone who took a horrendous situation and, through hope and determination, turned it into skills for her life that she has passed on to others. Challenges are inevitable, but we decide if we're going to learn something from the experience. As Eva discovered, the joy of learning is being able to share our story. As we continue to navigate our own lives, let's share our stories about how we are growing and building hope. As Emily Dickinson writes, "Hope is the thing with feathers that perches in the soul and sings the tune without the words and never stops at all."[30] Wishing you a hope filled day.

ON THE HOT SEAT

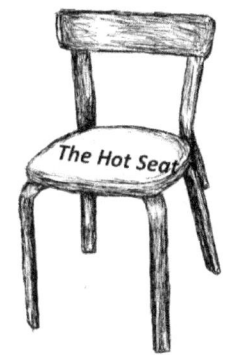

The Hot Seat

In the summer when the car has been sitting in the sun too long it's difficult to sit on the upholstery because it's overheated and far from comfortable. Sometimes it can't be sat on and the car door must be left open until the outside breeze cools the upholstery. Nobody likes an overheated seat. The topic here, however, is about a different kind of hot seat - the hot seat of criticism which can be emotionally charged and very uncomfortable. Criticism is a form of judgement or evaluation, and if it's given by someone who truly wants to help us it's done kindly and becomes constructive. We all make decisions during our day that affect other people which means we will receive feedback about our choices. When we're on the hot seat we want to handle criticism like a pro, so here are a few ideas for doing that so we cool things down and keep our inner peace intact.

Perhaps the hardest thing to do is to take a deep breath and remain calm when what we really want to do is defend ourself. Yes, we need to respond, but let's let go of our ego and not take anything personally (I know this is hard) because if we don't, we could spend our whole life being offended. Let's not get stuck on who's right or wrong. This is the time to silence our inner "know-it-all". Keeping our cool will save us from saying or doing something we'll later regret.

It's also important to look at who is doing the criticizing. If it's someone we trust and respect then we can listen carefully to determine what rings true. Sometimes critics see our blind spots, so if we look for the nugget of truth in whatever is being said and use it as an opportunity for growth, we've handled criticism like a pro. If it's someone who thrives on tearing others down than cut them off – rudeness, insults and abuse are not acceptable. This is destructive criticism. Avoid these people even if they are a longtime friend or family member. Let's be selective about what we take on board.

The hot seat helps us develop the skill of defining our differences. It's appropriate to be specific about how we may see something differently. Being overly accommodating to avoid conflict doesn't help because peace at any cost is self-destructive. Here's an old saying that rings true, "When you dim your light to please others, the whole world gets darker." Timing is essential to being heard so we may need to save what we want to say for another conversation when receptivity is higher. Remember, the response of the other person is not in our control.

No matter what aspect of our life the comments are about, whenever we're given rough feedback let's give ourself time to process what's been said so we can respond thoughtfully. We can ask questions and request specific examples for clarity. With an open mind we can experience new ways of thinking and feeling which may take some practice. This will create something positive out of being on the hot seat. Appreciation can be expressed for the critique acknowledging the courage it took to share their feelings. Taking time to apologize for whatever our part of the problem is will work the miracle of turning combat into collaboration.

Sometimes what feels the worst can turn out to be the best. As Byron Katie writes in her book **A Mind At Home With Itself**, "Criticism is the greatest gift you can receive if self-realization is what you're interested in."[31] She reminds us that we choose our feelings so no one can hurt us without our permission. When we bring our best selves to the hot seat we create an environment for growth, keep our peace of mind, and avoid being a victim. When handled well, the discomfort of the hot seat does have its rewards as we see deeper into 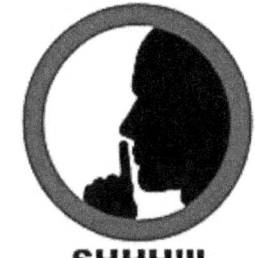 ourself and others. With a little practice we can handle the hot seat like a pro.

SAYING MORE BY TALKING LESS

Silence has a power all its own. When we're silent we're not being unresponsive, instead we're allowing our thought process and intuition to sort things out before we speak. Silence is not a weakness or a refusal to see a problem, it's harnessing our inner calm in a heated moment so we don't say things we later regret. Silence is not ignorance of a situation and calmness is not acceptance of an injustice. Silence and calmness are signs of strength and courage and both are needed before any action is taken.

Some people are so uncomfortable with silence that they continue to talk even if they have nothing meaningful to say. They not only stress the people around them but completely miss the gifts silence has to offer. I appreciate a person who knows the power of silence because, when used with intention, it's a communication superpower. When I was teaching high school, I used the practice of silence in the classroom. If I was quiet, students immediately knew to pay attention – no words or raised voice needed. A silent stare was a reminder to someone who had momentarily forgotten our agreed upon class rules.

Let's look at some of the gifts of silence. The Dalai Lama wrote, "When you talk you are only repeating what you already know. But if you listen, you may learn something new."[32] Silence can be the doorway to wisdom. When we give our full attention to whoever is speaking, we'll better understand their message and our reaction to it.

Research indicates active listeners create stronger relationships built on connection and trust. Silence enhances observation skills so we are aware of our surroundings and understand the situation better. It allows us to put ourself in the other person's shoes which improves our conflict resolution skills.

Silence gives us time for reflection and promotes healing when we take time to go deep within ourself. Luminita D. Saviuc writes, "Silence is a precious gift we give ourselves. In that space between our words, not only do we find ourselves, but we can also hear our own heart talking to us, our soul and intuition."[33]

When we're quiet we can concentrate our focus which promotes clarity and enhances decision making skills. This is especially helpful when a nasty social media post arrives that we completely disagree with. Rather than respond with more anger, let's give it the silent treatment and stop that negative energy. People who are dealing with loss or illness just want to be heard, and empathetic listening is sometimes all that is needed. Unwanted advice only adds more stress to the situation.

Research also shows that quieter people are better at managing their emotions so knee jerk reactions are avoided and composure is maintained, even in difficult situations. Resilience is also increased. Quiet people can be better communicators because their thoughtful approach means their words clearly convey their message. They are also more flexible in new situations.

Sometimes silence is more powerful than words and inevitably can never be misquoted. It helps to remember that words are sacred and need to be carefully chosen. Also, let's remember silence is sacred. So, let's use words when we have something valuable to say and learn the power of saying more by talking less. As Abraham Lincoln once said, "It's better to be thought a fool than to open your mouth and remove all 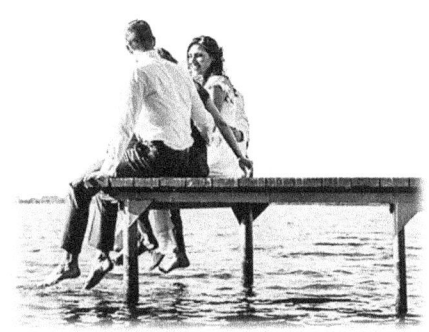 doubt."[34] The key is balance between silence and speaking. Let's try more listening and less talking and see what happens. This communication superpower is at our disposal.

THE ART OF LAZINESS

Laziness is often considered a flaw in human behavior. Growing up I was told idle hands would get into trouble, so keeping busy was applauded. This is not about people who refuse to contribute in any way, which is unhealthy laziness. This is about healthy laziness that promotes balance. The art of laziness is the ability to rethink productivity, create boundaries, practice flexibility, take breaks, and focus on what is most important.

A change in the way we think about busy days and relaxation may be overdue, because science is proving laziness is actually good for us. Science tells us that when we're relaxed, we're more innovative, we focus better, and creativity is higher. Bill Gates writes, "I will always choose a lazy person to do a difficult job, because a lazy person will find an easy way to do it."[35] This means a healthy laziness can make us more effective and efficient.

Think about historic Ben Franklin, who is thought of as a hard-working person. Here is how he describes himself, "I'm the laziest person in the world. I invented all those things to save myself from toil."[36] Perhaps there is some natural laziness in all of us, otherwise we wouldn't have computers, microwaves, or remote controls.

Laziness improves our health by lowering blood pressure. An afternoon nap reduces stress and refreshes both body and mind. Stress induced inflammation is lowered which produces a calming effect on skin conditions like psoriasis, eczema and rosacea. Relaxing improves our night time sleep so we wake with improved memory, and sharper thinking skills. Science now supports that keeping fit can be achieved with short, intense workouts. Strategic laziness helps our minds to wander freely, allowing the most insightful ideas to emerge. It's also a sure way to prevent burnout.

Laziness helps our emotional intelligence because it gives us time to reflect, and become more self-aware. When needed, it helps us apologize more effectively. We also become more sensitive to social cues from other people, so we see their emotional state more accurately. This improves our ability to create needed boundaries, enhance communication, and clarify problems. Drama is avoided because lazy people don't want to spend time gossiping or arguing. Healthy laziness improves relationships.

Our focus is improved with laziness because our concentration is on eliminating irrelevant activities, and simplifying our day. We relieve ourself from the tyranny of the urgent, so only what is vital gets attention. There's no need to micromanage anything because a relaxed person knows how to either let it go, or delegate. Instead of an insatiable need to stay busy, downtime is embraced, creating time for reflection and a deeper appreciation of the present moment.

Chris Bailey, author of **Hyperfocus**, writes, "I don't mean laziness in the sense of filling each moment with mindless distraction. I mean proper idleness when we choose to do nothing."[37] Distractions are everywhere, but we can choose to ignore them and put our physical and mental feet up. When we do this, we restore our energy, unnecessary tasks disappear, we connect with our guiding intuition, and practice flexibility.

Whatever is going on in our life, our worth is not dependent on how many tasks we do each day. We can actually accomplish more by doing less. This applies to whatever stage of life we're in. And it's true even if our activities are limited because of illness, or we're the caregiver keeping a household together. When we focus on the essential, we can let everything else go. It's a balanced day that promotes health on all levels. I'm suggesting we give ourselves daily permission to practice the art of laziness, so we can go with the flow instead of getting stuck in stress. Jeff Foster in his poem *Let Yourself Rest* writes, "Feel the fullness of the emptiness, the vastness of the silence, the sheer life in your unproductive moments. Time does not always have to be filled. You are enough, simply in your being."[38]

THE POWERFUL GIFT OF CHOICE

Our days are filled with choices,
conscious and unconscious, small and
large, that enable us to accept what we are presently experiencing, and
act with courage to create needed changes. Instead of being a victim of
circumstance, we can choose to be the creator of our circumstances. This
is about more than what we eat, wear, or read. This is about turning our
lives into a miraculous journey that fosters loving relationships, inner
peace, and personal fulfillment no matter what our circumstances may
be.

Remember the definition of insanity is doing what we've always done,
but expecting different results. This plays out when we are stuck in an
unconscious pattern of behavior that takes difficult challenges, and only
addresses the outward circumstances. We miss the opportunity for a
different outcome. This isn't where change takes place. Effective, lasting,
change begins on the inside - it's an inside out approach to life.

An honest look within will reveal any self-limiting, or self-sabotaging
beliefs we may have carried with us for years. This affects how we view
the circumstances of our lives. Whatever we believe we attract to
ourselves. When we use our power of choice to let go of self-critical
beliefs, we enhance and elevate our life experiences into more rewarding
relationships, and inner harmony. Remember, it isn't what happens to us
that matters, it's the choices we make that transform our lives. Every
circumstance, no matter how difficult, is an opportunity for us to evolve
from confusion into peace, from frustration to fulfillment.

As we learn how to most effectively use our power of choice, let's
remember that we are all on an individual development continuum.

Being patient and compassionate with each other is essential. Resisting the urge to judge ourselves or others is also essential. I don't know about you, but I'm more critical of myself then I am of anyone else, and some days I need to remind myself to stop being hard on myself, and choose to be kind instead. When we feel the urge to be critical of ourselves or others, let's remind ourselves that we are doing our best. We don't know the other person's story, or how limited their options may be. This is the time to choose to be affirming and supportive.

Using our powerful gift of choice, we can turn our lives into an incredible journey that undoes limits, and enhances healing love and inner contentment. We awaken and know our negative experiences do not define us. We awaken and know we can choose not to be afraid as well. We awaken and know love is stronger than fear. We awaken and choose to be confident, courageous, kind, and content. We awaken and know that even a serious illness or the passing of a loved one does not limit our inner peace. We awaken and know that we can choose what is right for us.

Sometimes it's difficult to see, but we all have access to the power of choice and the gifts it brings. We can choose to align ourselves with spiritual wisdom, and we can choose to protect ourselves from people who are unsupportive or critical. When we know what empowers us, we can choose to stay focused on that. Wayne Dyer writes, "Be miserable. Or motivate yourself. Whatever has to be done, it's always your choice."[39] Let's take this powerful gift and use it to enhance our own lives, so we open ourselves to the miracles around and within us. The powerful gift of choice is always ours.

THE POWER OF PERSEVERANCE

The movie "Ride Like a Girl" tells the story of Michelle Payne.[40] She was born in Australia, in 1985, the youngest of ten children. Her father, Paddy Payne was a race horse trainer. When Michelle was six months old, her mother had a fatal car accident leaving Paddy with ten children, and a business to run. The children grew up taking care of their race horses and stables in between going to school. Paddy trained all of his children to ride and eight out of the ten became jockeys participating in competitions.

Michelle had the greatest passion for racing of all the children and announced, at age seven, that she was going to win The Melbourne Cup. She chafed under her father's training, always wanting to do more than he thought she was ready for. After a major argument she stepped out on her own to enter the male dominated world of jockeys. She was laughed at, ridiculed, and told to go home. She stayed, continued to enter races, and even though she did poorly in early competition, continued to learn on the job. In 2004 she fell during a race, and her injuries were so severe she was told she might not walk again, much less ride competitively.

After a year of hard therapeutic work, Michelle, barely able to climb on her horse, slowly started riding again. She was determined to follow her racing dream, and willing to do the hard work to make that happen. Gradually she began competing with her father's voice in her head reminding her to "always look for the opening and take it when it happens." Her persistence paid off and she began winning races until she qualified to run in the most prestigious race in Australia – The Melbourne Cup. In 2015, she was a relatively unknown rider on an unknown horse, so the odds of her winning were set at impossible, or one hundred to one. As the race progressed to the final push toward the finish line, she saw the opening her father had talked about, slipped into it, pulled ahead and became the first female jockey to win the Melbourne Cup.

It was perseverance that kept her training through tensions with her father, injuries, prejudice, and moments of discouragement. Perseverance is the ability to keep going despite obstacles, setbacks, or challenges. It's the staying power to exert effort until the goal or dream is achieved. It's the ability to keep going one step at a time when the finish line is nowhere in sight. People who persevere know hardships and failure at some point along the way but, with clear vision, they keep their goal in sight.

Here are a few ideas for harnessing the power of perseverance. First, we need to be clear about what we want to achieve, including ideas on how to get there. Then, when setbacks happen we need to break down the problem into small steps so it isn't overwhelming. People who persevere ask for help when they need it. They actively seek advice, support, and encouragement when times get tough. They are hopeful and optimistic about finding solutions. Then we can take the Dhali Larma's attitude which is, "If there is a solution to the problem then don't waste time worrying about it. If there is **no** solution to the problem then don't waste time worrying about it."[41]

Taking care of ourselves is essential to any success so we need to pay attention to diet, exercise, rest, social contacts, and staying hydrated. Perseverance can flourish when we keep ourselves encouraged by eliminating negative self-talk, reading inspiring stories, and participating in support groups. We must avoid comparing ourselves to others, knowing each of us has our own individual journey, with its own timeline.

We harness the power of perseverance when we do what brings us joy. In Joseph Campbell's words, "Find a place inside where there's joy, and the joy will burn out the pain."[42] Showing appreciation to others through acts of kindness and expressing gratitude are two powerful ways to increase joy and fuel perseverance. Let's remember that people who love and support us are a treasure.

Perseverance through challenges makes us stronger and more confident in our problem solving. It's perseverance in the tough times that heightens our appreciation of everyday life. Through perseverance we learn to build resilience and accomplish more with renewed wisdom. With the power of perseverance, we become more focused in decision making and clarify exactly what we want. The more we practice the better we become at it, so every small accomplishment is to be appreciated. Perseverance is an ongoing process so let's keep each other encouraged. Like Michelle, we can take whatever life gives us and continue to follow our dream. In the words of Abraham Lincoln, "The best thing about the future is that it only comes one day at a time." [43] We can handle that.

WHAT GEAR AM I IN?

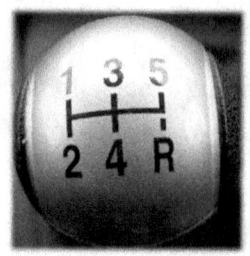

We all know life is full of change. What we focus on determines how well we manage to navigate our personal journey. Major challenges make it hard for even the most optimistic among us to stay positive. Of course, we need to take any world event seriously, but if we stay focused on calamity, our thoughts and actions may become fearful and counterproductive.

While it's important to identify danger and respond appropriately, it is also important to know when to shift gears. My husband and I have increased our biking recently, and I began thinking about the significance of gears. If we are riding a bike with a selection of gears, we know all the gears are important. The last thing we want to do is get stuck in a gear ineffective for the terrain we're riding over. If we're going uphill, we need to shift to a lower gear so we can make the climb without exhausting ourselves. Without switching gears, we may fold half way up the hill, unable to finish the climb.

Emotionally we need to be able to switch gears so we don't get stuck in a fearful place, unable to make productive decisions. Being positive is not naive or simplistic, nor does it mean ignoring life's challenges. What it does mean is putting yourself in the driver's seat, with the "life bicycle" in the right gear, so life can be navigated with the help of open-minded thinking. It means choosing to be resilient which leads to hope, serenity, and gratitude.

Here are a few ideas for staying in the right gear despite difficult circumstances. While we limit our intake of daily bad news to help foster positivity, let's remember past difficult experiences that were major life disrupter s can be viewed positively. We did handle those unforeseen challenges then, and we can do it now. We are resilient. Positivity helps us stay in the right gear and positivity builds when we do random acts of kindness. It's fun to send a note of thanks to a friend or colleague. Watch the smiles on the faces of grocery store employees, postal workers, and pharmacists when we say a verbal "thank you" for their services.

I'm sending our grandson books from his favorite author, through Amazon, to add some fun after school work is completed. He loves knowing more books are coming. My husband sent a copy of his pilot's log to his cousin who flew with him to Alaska in a small plane. Together they fished the commercial salmon run many years ago. The two of them are thoroughly enjoying reliving the excitement of their youthful adventure. These small kindnesses build positive emotions and keep us in the "right gear" for managing tough terrain. We boost our spirits when we take time to notice all the people who are helping others right now. When we each do our part, we support and encourage each other.

We stay in the right gear when we invest in what is uplifting. This is the time for our favorite inspirational books, music, and people's stories of courage. We need to keep ourselves connected to people who know how to stay in the "right gear", who love us and offer healthy support. Recently, my husband and I met eight other people in a park and spent a couple of hours sitting in the shade sipping, and snacking. We talked about what was the best and what was the hardest part about our personal challenges. There was plenty of support and laughter which made it meaningful, rewarding and oh so uplifting!

William Arruda writes, "In times of constant negative messaging, you need an antidote so that you can keep your positive attitude and march forward with determination and hope. Be deliberate in activities that are positive, heartwarming, stress reducing and laughter inducing."[44] Sounds like excellent advice for selecting the "right gear" to navigate whatever life brings. Let's keep pedaling together.

Chapter 6 – Nurturing Relationships

CELEBRATING OUR DIVERSITY WITH UNITY

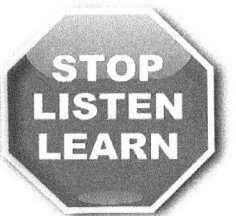

Our universe is characterized by much diversity with galaxies of stars, comets and planets, instead of just one type of each. An orchestra is made up of an assortment of instruments, not just violins. Our bodies are made up of multiple organs that each preform unique functions. It's the diversity of many organs working together that make it complete and able to function optimally. We humans are meant to be an array of differences so we can work together to experience functioning optimally.

Unless we're Native American, we are immigrants bringing our assortment of cultural gifts to the USA, for instance. From India comes Chef Padma Lakshmi[1] who specializes in cuisine from immigrant and indigenous people. Her work with immigrants, women's rights, and the American Civil Liberties Union inspired her to create a cookbook, and a Television show, featuring food from across our country that reflect different cultures, and tell people's ethnic stories. She reminds us that there's no such thing as an "all-American food" unless it is Native American. She's an example of someone celebrating cultural diversity that highlights our common bond in food preperation.

This next example comes from my husband's career in aviation, and shows the importance of male/female cooperation. On April 28, 1988, Aloha Flight 243 (a Boeing 737) lost a large section off the top of the aircraft while in flight.[2] In the cockpit were Captain Robert Schornstheimer, and 1st Officer Madeline Tompkins and both pilots immediately went into crisis aircraft management. This was such a unique emergency they could not navigate it using only the Flight Operations Manual. Together they problem solved their way to a successful landing with only

1 death. As their crisis management style was studied, it became evident that the success of their working together lay in both accepting and using both the masculine and feminine perspective while decision making. Since that event, an intense and ongoing study has revealed that the optimal combination in a cockpit is to have both male and female present. Such diversity is our strength when we work together in this way.

My husband and I have had opportunities for travel that have opened our hearts to other parts of the world, and given us lessons in cultural differences that enriched our lives. It's helpful to know that travel isn't necessary for cultural experiences; it can happen right here if we're willing to stretch ourselves out of the familiar. We can travel through our Smart TV channels to almost any country in the world, and discover how important all people's stories are to the health and well-being of our human race. Trying international cuisine is fun, as is listening to music with ethnic roots. Traditional folk tales from around the world have been part of many of our childhoods. Museums are dedicated to foster cultural experiences but, if going in person isn't possible, we can go online and find numerous ethnic galleries to view. We can also visit a church we don't normally attend to learn about different religions. Seeing the world through the eyes of another culture is life changing, and often reveals we are more alike than different.

Delores Penn wrote, "Presently our country is going through some difficult times. We can say to ourselves that it doesn't have anything to do with me and my beliefs, or we can stop, listen, and learn."[3] This is definitely the time to "stop, listen, and learn!" It might be hard and uncomfortable getting started, but it's time to remember that our worth is about who we are. It's time to practice respect for our differences, and it's time to discover more of our commonalities.

The essence of our physical world is tremendous diversity, and we as humans can reflect that in interdependence, compassionate acts , cooperation, sharing and caring. There is room for every point of view, culture, race, and language. Our differences aren't meant for separation; they represent the beauty found in our unity. Change begins within each one of us when we "stop, listen, and learn." Let's celebrate our diversity with equality, equity and cooperation in a way that compliments each other. Diversity is worth celebrating when we do it in unity.

L. R. Knost writes, "Do not be dismayed by the brokenness of the world. All things break. And all things can be mended. Not with time, as they say, but with intention. So go, love intentionally, extravagantly, unconditionally. The broken world waits in darkness for the light that is you."[4]

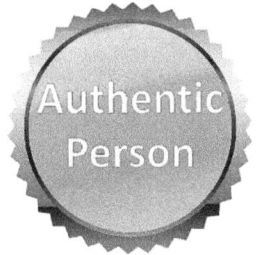

COME AS YOU ARE

It's tempting to identify ourselves by our job title, financial status, personal circumstances, physical fitness, or affiliations. Where does that leave us when our marriage implodes, we lose our job or face a serious health diagnosis? This is about being authentic, and our authentic self is not defined by any of those categories. Our uniqueness is a combination of our genetic gifts along with our life experiences. We are truly ourself when we stop being a chameleon and show up with our integrity and the gifts that are uniquely ours to share. E. E. Cummings wrote, "It takes courage to grow up and become who you really are."[5]

Have you ever had the experience of making a decision based on what other people will think instead of what is right for you? Many of us have had to go against family expectations when choosing a career, partner, or place to live. My husband did not join his dad's business because it wasn't right for him. When I was younger, I allowed pressure from others to influence a decision I made that violated my values. I felt awful afterwards. It was an important lesson and I didn't allow that to happen again.

Authenticity can show up in small events too. Yesterday I was in a clothing store and witnessed this. Three women were shopping together but only one was buying. The two women not buying were busy telling the other one what to try on, what they liked and what she should purchase. The woman buying did exactly as she was told and walked out of the store being congratulated on making a good decision. The buyer was never asked what she liked, what made her feel good or what reflected who she was. She dressed to satisfy her friends.

Much as we would like a shortcut to authenticity, there isn't one. Coming as we are to any situation requires inner honesty and commitment. It starts with one small decision after another that supports what is most important to us. Brené Brown wrote, "Authenticity is the daily practice of letting go of who we think we're supposed to be and embracing who we are."[6]

If we're going to come as we are, we can start by accepting ourselves and letting go of other people's business and their approval. Living in our own truth means we create a daily practice of saying no to anything that doesn't support who we are. We can say no to a draining social engagement or a project that isn't right for us. We have the courage to set boundaries.

Part of being authentic is owning our mistakes, forgiving ourself, and loving ourself by embracing our imperfections. Christine Carter writes, "Loving and accepting ourselves – and all of our flaws, including our anger and fear and sadness and pettiness – is, in the end, the only thing that enables us to be authentic. It is also the greatest gift we can give ourselves. It is the reason that authenticity makes us happier and healthier and more connected to those around us."[7]

Coming as we are requires stepping out of our comfort zone. We may experience criticism, but when we live an inauthentic life everything that we're keeping inside festers leading to anxiety, depression, anger, blame and resentment. We can expand our integrity by inviting moments of solitude into our day so we disconnect from distracting outside voices. These voices come from a culture that prioritizes what we do instead of who we are. We can be the voice of support to others who are choosing to be themselves, the voice of love when fear surrounds us, and the voice of encouragement for taking care of body, mind and spirit.

There are important reasons for living true to ourself. We live with more vitality because there is less inner conflict. Because we have less inner conflict, we'll have more insights into what motivates us, and this in turn will help us be more tolerant and understanding of others. If we're grounded in our authentic inner self, we're more able to resist social pressures resulting in better decision making. Let's come as we are wherever we go. What is needed is our authenticity.

CONNECTING THROUGH COMPASSION

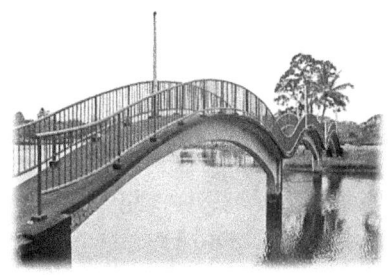

Nurturing our connections is always important, but current events and personal challenges can make this even more critical. Isolation and polarized views are challenging our connection to compassion for both ourself and others. Our differences don't need to divide us if we're willing to build bridges. Brené Brown writes in her book **Braving the Wilderness**, "People are hard to hate close up. Move in."[8] Moving in is building a bridge.

We all have people in our lives who see the world through a different lens than we do, or have opposing views. If we're willing to stop labeling others as good or bad, right or wrong, and instead allow for differences, we can meet in the middle with out-stretched hands instead of clenched fists. Compassion doesn't mean people can get away with hurting others, but it does separate the behavior from the person. When we connect through a compassionate bridge, we acknowledge we are all part of the human family.

The following quote is by Pema Chodron, "Compassion is not a relationship between the healer and wounded. It's a relationship between equals. Only when we know our darkness well, can we be present with the darkness of others. Compassion becomes real when we recognize our shared humanity."[9]

To move in and build bridges of compassion, we first need to start by being compassionate to ourself. We acknowledge our successes, forgive our mistakes, and focus on our strengths instead of giving ourself a diet of criticism. We acknowledge the places where we're wounded, and promote our own healing. Prioritizing self-compassion means we address our needs when they're small, so they don't become overwhelming. It helps to breathe deeply, slow down, make decisions mindfully, and get plenty of sleep. And let's acknowledge our small successes throughout the day. When we're patient and kind to ourself, we'll radiate a positive, inclusive energy.

We build bridges by the way we communicate both verbally and nonverbally. Let's remember that words are powerful, and we need to choose them carefully so we express compassion, not judgement. People have a variety of views and values that have been affected by their environment, early parenting, and life experiences. There are many reasons why we are the way we are. When we bring a loving attitude to the present moment, our words become supportive and encouraging while setting boundaries. Thus, lets us move in and connect. Remember that compassion does not mean we need to stay in toxic relationships.

Showing compassion nonverbally starts when we turn our smartphone to airplane mode, so the person we're with has our complete attention. Giving our true presence is a powerful gift. To do that we turn toward the speaker, give them eye contact, and quietly listen. It can be incredibly healing when both tears and laughter are shared. These are small acts that build strong bridges.

Another way to move in is through showing kindness. Wherever we are, whatever we're doing, being kind is contagious, so one act begins the ripple effect. We are truly practicing kindness when we do kind acts without expecting anything in return. An unexpected kindness can comfort and encourage someone having a hard day. It's the compassionate connection with a kind presence that lifts the spirits of everyone involved.

Respecting a person's privacy is another way to move in and build bridges. Whenever something intimate is shared, it needs to stay between the people involved. Compassion does not gossip. And when someone isn't ready to talk about the hard stuff, we can affirm our support by simply being a caring presence.

Remembering our common humanity is connecting through compassion in a powerful way. What we choose to focus on affects our perspective. When we encourage each other in healthy self-care, thoughtful communication, kindness, and respect, we bridge our differences and nurture each other. Let's remember we're all part of the human family and need each other.

DEEP LISTENING

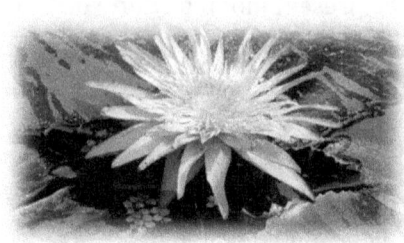

"Mom, do you have time for a visit?" my son said over the phone. He is mostly home bound recovering from extensive lower leg and foot surgery. "Of course – what's on your mind?" I replied. He had been pondering his life journey, seeing in retrospect what could not be seen in the immediacy of events. While using this surgical recovery time to thoughtfully sort through how his past brought him to where he is now, he had gained new perspective and clarity. He wanted to share this with me. All he wanted was for me to listen to what he had to say – no advice or lengthy comments – just listen. He had my willing and undivided attention. When he was done, he thanked me for treating what he had to say with openness and respect, and without judgement. Knowing he was heard was the basis for his gratitude at the end of our conversation. And I knew his heartfelt sharing was a bonding, healing gift for both of us.

If we want to listen on a deep level, we need to prepare by detaching from our own agenda. Mark Nepo has this to say about deep listening, "Before we can truly listen, we must exhaust ourselves of our assumptions. In truth, if we are ever to glimpse the world outside the stubborn certainty of our minds, we have to put down our ready answer to everything."[10] This means resisting the impulse to dip into our storehouse of opinions to defend our point of view

Offering a peaceful, loving, listening presence is one of the most meaningful ways to take care of our relationships. Linda Popov puts it this way, "Our capacity to be fully present to each other in the moment is the single most powerful way to sustain love and show that we cherish one another. It is the greatest gift we have to give anyone. When we are present, we engage in each other's lives, take each other seriously, and meet one another with full, focused attention, with discernment and understanding."[11] If a listening presence is a conduit of love, then it is indeed powerful.

I suspect we have all experienced of talking to someone and knowing their attention was somewhere else. We know when it's happening – no eye contact, flippant remarks, multitasking - and how it feels to be dismissed, as though we were unworthy of someone else's time. Relationships wither when we stop meaningful listening.

If we want to confirm our commitment to the people we love, we need to consciously practice undistracted attention, show interest, maintain eye contact, and affirm their importance. Our compassion also shows when we listen in receptive silence which creates a safe space for others to speak freely. When we offer receptive, caring silence along with compassion, we affirm that we're ready to hear someone else's story. Giving the gift of receptivity and nonjudgmental attention invites soul sharing.

Being a caring listener does not include rescuing or fixing. As women, we often take on the role of caregiver. If we decide to become the emotions police, we will be trying to keep everyone around us "happy". It's an impossible task that results in frustration for all involved. We can genuinely care by hearing their story, without sliding into fixing the situation.

The gift of being a deep listener invites each of us to help the other in slowly unwrapping our cocoon, to release the beauty hidden within. That is the power of deep listening!

THE POWER OF PATIENCE

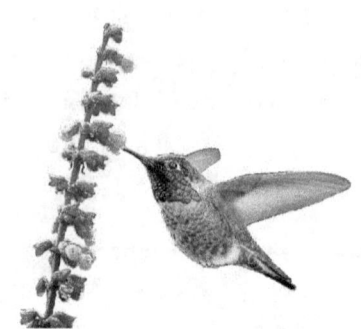

Patience is a necessary virtue for
life management that lowers
stress, and leads to decisions
based on thoughtfulness, and
clarity. It is a way of being that
improves our experiences, calms our frustrations, and transforms
challenges into growth. Patience is a powerful practice that can enhance
every aspect of our life.

We all have plenty of elements in our lives that could keep us in a crazy,
frustrated, victimized state, but that is an awful place to live. In that state
we often try to force an outcome that doesn't work because our attitude,
thinking, and behavior lack calmness, and clear thought. Yes, it's
upsetting when we accidentally delete a computer file, see politicians and
police behaving badly, or experience delayed medical test results, but
losing our cool won't help. Impatience only makes things worse by
keeping stress levels high.

Let's remember patience doesn't mean passivity or resignation – it
means power. It's the power of knowing when to wait and when to act.
It's the power that comes with being mindful, focused, and
compassionate. It's the power to choose how we will handle everything
from a major crisis to daily hassles, with healthy boundaries, and non-
hostile behavior. Patience allows us to feel all the emotions that go with
life's challenges, while trusting the process we're in to take us where we
most need to go, whether we understand it or not.

As with any virtue, practice is needed, so here are a few suggestions for
developing the power of patience. Let's remember that even though

choosing patience can be difficult, especially when we want immediate changes, we can do hard things. We can start by breathing deeply which is calming, and moves us from tense thoughts to relaxing our body, which breaks the automatic stress response. Remember, what we focus on we attract, so let's be clear on what we want to invite into our life.

We practice patience when we take time to look at the big picture, and acknowledge that frustrating people and situations can be a source of personal growth. Asking ourself, "What do I need to change in myself to help this situation?" is a good place to start. Until we address our part in the scenario, we can't expect other people to address theirs. We become more patient when we accept what is, even though we may not like or agree with what is happening. When we stop fighting with the way things are, we open ourself up to creative problem solving and the chance for peaceful resolutions.

Patience grows when we practice gratitude, appreciate life, and see beauty around us. Slowing down gives us time to value the richness of life, and patience allows time for things to work themselves out. Rather than insisting on a quick fix, we can choose to wait until we really know what to do next. If we are patient, it will come naturally and harmoniously, and we will feel empowered because we are.

When we are kind to ourself, our patience grows. Let's recognize our strengths, as well as our faults, and welcome areas of weakness as places for growth. One tool for personal growth is to write thoughts down on paper, which lets us examine them with clearer perspective. We can see what's unhealthy and holding us back, so needed adjustments can be made. Many of us have given our kids a "time out" to reconsider behavior – sometimes we need to give ourself a "time out" so our bodies and brains calm down.

Patience comes when we recognize our Higher Power, so we never need to feel we are handling life alone. Spiritual practices strengthen our ability to hear our inner intuition, which opens us up to guidance. We can live in the knowledge that all is well, despite outward appearances. This helps us patiently let go of the need to be perfect, have all the answers, and be the one in control. This is where we find love for ourselves and others, and respect for the growth process we are all in together. When the power of patience is combined with love, the results can be life changing.

If you're like me, in one of those times when I wish I had the answers, but doesn't, it helps to remember what Rainer Maria Rilke said, "Be patient toward all that is unresolved in your heart and try to love the questions themselves. Do not now seek the answers, which cannot be given you because you would not be able to live them. And the point is to live everything. Live the questions."[12] Patience gives us the power to live the questions. And patience can prepare us to learn the lessons we need to learn for changes to happen when the time is right. Blocks will be removed as things get worked out in ourselves and others, so our job is to relax and trust. The power of patience gives us choices that can change even the most difficult situation. Let's not give this power away to knee jerk reactions - instead let's embrace the transformative power inherent in patience.

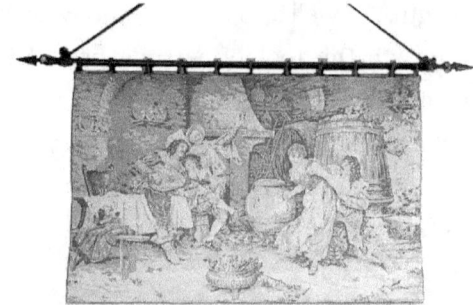

THE TAPESTRY OF LIFE

Threads have a long history of telling personal stories. History tells us that textiles were the language of the French who specialized in visual messaging through their clothing and artwork, choosing colors that declared allegiances and personal relationships. Political and personal statements were stitched into the folds of a skirt or even drapes on the windows. Threads stated one's lineage and wealth.

Quilt threads have a long history of telling the stories of families. My mother made me a double wedding ring quilt as a gift when I was married. It's the quilt that celebrates unity. Other quilts tell stories of traveling to new places, building a home, celebrating the birth of a child or remembering someone who has passed on. My sister-in-law made a quilt to tell the story of her recovery from breast cancer. Yarn threads are used to create prayer shawls to support and encourage women with cancer.

Having personally participated in needlepoint, knitting, embroidery, and sewing everything from clothes to quilts, I have seen threads of every color, weight and style come together beautifully after originally looking like an unorganized mess. Sometimes the back of a project is a mess with dropped stitches, knots, crisscrossing threads and frayed edges. It's a little like life. Our life can be looked at as a tapestry made up of our choices, conversations, unexpected events and the encounters we have with various people.

There are threads of revelation and inspiration, harmony and discord, togetherness and separateness, unexpected events and family traditions. Not only do we add to our own threads, but every person we have encountered since birth has added a thread to us and us to them. We're all interconnected. Our unique contribution is part of a larger tapestry that tells the story of all of us.

Today, each of us is an example of the thousands of threads that have come together rich with meaning because of our life experiences. It can be hard to see the big picture when we're in the middle of a difficult time. Sometimes all we see is knotted and frayed threads that look like they're ready to break. This is when we need to be present with our emotions, which represent another thread. When we need to rest and be quiet, our threads are still weaving because we're nurturing ourself. Every thread has its purpose and adds to the value of our tapestry.

This is a good time to remind ourself that life, like tapestry, is made up of different colors both light and dark. A full, vibrant life contains every color. It's the dark colors and shadows that create perspective and depth for the lighter colors in a tapestry. Our dark experiences give us perspective and depth as well. When our life threads get dark, we need to give ourself compassion and not lose sight of the big picture. Wayne Dyer wrote, "As I look back on the entire tapestry of my life, I can see from the perspective of the present moment that every aspect of my life was necessary and perfect. Each step actually led to a higher place, even though these steps often felt like obstacles or painful experiences."[13]

Have you ever looked on the back of a piece of needlepoint or tapestry? It's a confusing mess that makes no sense. Sometimes it feels like we're living in that kind of chaos. Only when we turn it over is the beauty of the picture revealed and it finally does make sense. The gorgeous patterns show our Higher Power is an accomplished artist that we can trust.

Our future involves new threads with everchanging colors. We are defining who we choose to be by weaving our tapestries from our guiding principles. Steven Covey wrote, "Principles are deep fundamental truths…. lightly interwoven threads running with exactness, consistence, beauty and strength through the fabric of life."[14] Our life is a tapestry and every moment adds threads to the masterpiece of our legacy. The beautifully intricate pattern that is ours is made of personal stories. Our unique stories need to be shared because we add to each other's woven art. Let's support and encourage each other, and embrace every thread knowing it is all part of the magnificent tapestry of who we all are.

VITAMIN F: FORGIVENESS AND FREEDOM

Vitamins have the capacity of enhancing our health so we can function optimally. But we need more than traditional vitamins to be at our best, so let's look at another ingredient that affects our health. I've taken the liberty to call forgiveness "Vitamin F" because it directly influences our well-being and relationships.

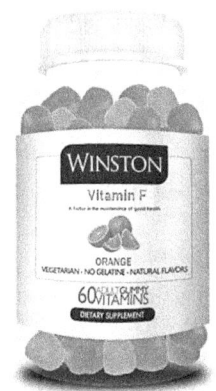

From personal experience I can verify the difference forgiveness makes. A while back I took a personal silent retreat and, in the middle of the night, suddenly woke and began remembering hurts from my past. I thought I had dealt with them, but obviously I needed to look at them again. Looking at them one more time, I realized every person involved had done what they had done out of ignorance, not intention. They just didn't know how to handle life differently. How could I fault them for that? Given their circumstances I might have behaved the same way. I fully released every incident and felt like a great weight had been lifted. The relief was tremendous and the result was my feeling light, free, and joyful.

Forgiveness is not about ignoring painful memories, or excusing hurtful behavior. *Psychology Today* describes forgiveness as "freeing ourselves from feelings of anger, resentment, and victimization, and ending with clarity about our values."[15] It's about having compassion and empathy for the person that caused the hurt, as well as for ourselves. Oprah

Winfrey describes forgiveness as, "Letting go of the belief that the past could have been any different."[16]

The process of forgiving and letting go is a catalyst for greater emotional, physical, mental, and spiritual health. As individuals get healthier, they affect their families, families affect communities, and communities affect the world. "Vitamin F" is powerful. Not using this "vitamin" has its costs because kept grievances result in anger, anxiety, frustration, depression, insomnia, addictions, and despair. Is this how we really want to live? There is a better alternative.

Ana Holub has written a book titled, **Forgive and Be Free**[17] in which she shares medical research coming from universities and medical centers studying forgiveness. She reiterates that anger and bitterness result in long-tern health problems, while forgiveness offers numerous health benefits. Here are a few of the health benefits of forgiveness from her book.

When we let go of anger from past grievances, our body responds with an even heart rate and lowered blood pressure. If we choose forgiveness instead of recycling anxious thoughts, we reduce stress hormones. We can also offer our concerns to our Higher Power which reduces emotional stress even further. Forgiveness reduces sudden hostile behaviors like road rage, or an urge to fight. When we let go of anger and bitterness we have more self-control, which gives us better anger management skills. Better anger management leads to a relaxed heart with a lower heart rate.

Often substance abuse masks underlying emotional pain. Forgiveness releases the pain and enables the forgiver to refocus on healthier behaviors. Forgiveness can lessen depression symptoms and lead the way to healing and compassion. When we learn to forgive others and ourselves, we have fewer anxiety symptoms, and are able to love ourselves more fully.

When we stop holding grudges, we are open to becoming closer to friends and family. That change also makes room for new relationships, and the relationships we create are healthier because there is less drama. Forgiveness brings us closer to Spirit which again enhances our well-being. When we offer up our fear, sadness, and pain, we receive peace, love and healing. This gives us improved psychological well-being so we feel calmer, happier, and able to live more harmoniously. With "Vitamin F" we lower our cortisol and boost our immune system.

Forgiveness is a choice we need to make daily. It uplifts our vibrational field and breaks patterns of fear. We forgive when we're ready and not a moment before, so let's go within and ask ourselves if we're ready to exchange our grievances for freedom and peace. When we give ourselves a regular dose of "Vitamin F", we improve our own health and the well-being of those around us. Robert Muller puts it this way, "To forgive is the highest, most beautiful form of love. In return, you will receive untold peace and happiness."[18] This is a "vitamin" worth taking!

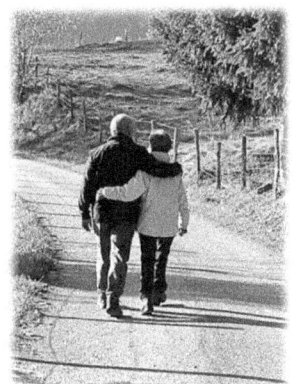

WALKING EACH OTHER HOME

We need each other. Time alone certainly gives us insights into knowing who we are, but there are some things about ourselves that can only be learned through interaction with others. It is being with other people, and experiencing life together, that allows us to know ourselves more fully. Together we provide transformational material for each other's journeys that can lead to becoming more of who we want to be. We are here to help each other gain clarity, so we can come home to ourselves in deep and profound ways. It was Ram Dass that wrote, "We're all just walking each other home."[19]

"Home is where the heart is" is a popular saying. Sometimes we lose connection with our heart and feel a deep yearning that can be hard to articulate. Finding our way back home to our heart is not done in isolation. Our lives have family, friends, colleagues, acquaintances, and even adversaries that become our travel companions on our journey home. Some of the people we walk with are lifelong companions, while others are with us for a limited time before our paths diverge.

Some short-lived relationships might feel like detours, but they are very much a part of our path. Certain people can create hardship in our life, however, their presence helps us clarify our priorities. When it comes to what we want to be and experience, it's just as important to know what we don't want as well as what we do want. This enables us to leave unhealthy relationships, seek a different job, choose a new doctor, or move to a new location. The pain of a difficult situation can be transformed when we are committed to learning and growing into our most authentic self.

Recently I read a story of a young woman whose husband showed her how to stand tall, to know who she was, and be true to herself. That became a beautiful and indelible part of who she is today. Entering into any relationship with intention and awareness enhances our ability to walk each other home. What if we looked at all the people we encounter daily, whether they are conscious of it or not, as playing a part in walking us home? What if we are playing a role in their homeward journey? How might we choose to be with someone if, at least for the moment, we are walking homeward side by side?

This is what we can do for each other. We say a soft word, give a gentle touch, embrace with a hug, listen with focus, and encourage with presence. We specialize in walking each other home again and again. The following is two stanzas in a song written by Stuart Stotts[20] about walking each other home.

Whatever story you may tell
To the world or to yourself
Right through heaven or through hell
We're walking each other home.
A word that's soft and a touch that's kind
An open heart and a patient mind
No one will be left behind
We're walking each other back home.

WORD POWER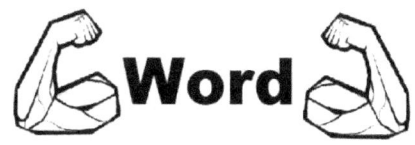

As a child when I was teased at school, I was told to say to myself, "Sticks and stones may break my bones, but words will never harm me." I didn't believe it. The cruel words hurt no matter how many times I repeated that sentence. That experience clarified my own desire to be a source of kind, not cruel words. On the positive side I remember as a young adult wondering if I had the potential to write anything more than letters and journals. A man I respected believed in me and my writing before I did, and that felt so supportive that I was encouraged to continue developing my skills. His words were the inspiration I needed.

Words carry the power to encourage, comfort and calm, as well as humiliate and destroy. We use them to describe what we believe about ourself and others. They affect our vision of the world and the quality of our life. Words shape our perceptions, form our beliefs, and drive our behavior. The parameters of our life are formed by the language that originates with our thoughts.

Words can uplift our personal energy or drag us down. Haven't we all been around someone who is so negative and full of complaints and demands that we can hardly wait to get away from them? Their words sap our energy so we feel depleted. Christiane Northrup, M.D. in her book **Dodging Energy Vampires**[21] literally calls these people "energy vampires" because they live off the energy of other people. This is why taking care of ourself and setting boundaries is essential. Then there are those lovely people who embrace us with encouraging words when we're struggling, withholding their judgement, and loving us just as we are. These people renew our energy and lift our spirits with their support. Word power is truly amazing.

How we talk to ourself is just as important as our language with others. Belittling our self in any way is harmful. And the more often we do this the more power it has over us because repetition increases validation. Politicians and product advertisers know all about this – used often enough repetition will trump the truth. This is why affirming statements like "I'm lovable or I'm able to solve this problem" are so important. A gift we can give ourself is to surround ourself with positive, uplifting words from ourself and others.

When we become mindful in our language choices, we avoid becoming the person who mindlessly gives voice to every thought and feeling dumping their minds contents without any regard to what they're saying. Selecting our words carefully and watching our tone of voice, we can speak our truth from a place of peace, compassion and respect. Betty Eadie wrote, "If we understood the power of our thoughts, we would guard them more closely. If we understood the awesome power of our words, we would prefer silence to almost anything negative. In our thoughts and words, we create our own weakness and our own strengths."[22]

We are social people created to interact with each other. Our brains are wired in what scientists call the "language network" which is the same area of our brain that also regulates our heart rate, adjusts glucose amounts and determines the flow of chemicals supporting our immune system. This means we affect each other's metabolisms. When talking with someone we care about, our breathing and heart rate will synchronize. This happens between infants and caregivers, singing choirs and yoga class participants. If we're with someone we don't like or trust, there is no harmony between our bodies and instead we create the disruption of our bodies smooth functioning. This is why people with a loving support system live longer.

We are the architects of our own word power, which is a sacred gift. Let's be selective in our word choices and careful in our delivery. Katherine Hurst Ph.D. wrote, "It is our words that provide a bold affirmation of our innermost thoughts. They are a confirmation to the world of how we see others, our lives and ourselves. It is this powerful affirmation that our words provide which enables our thoughts to manifest into reality."[23] Let's use our word power to nourish ourself, encourage others, and build a peace filled life and community.

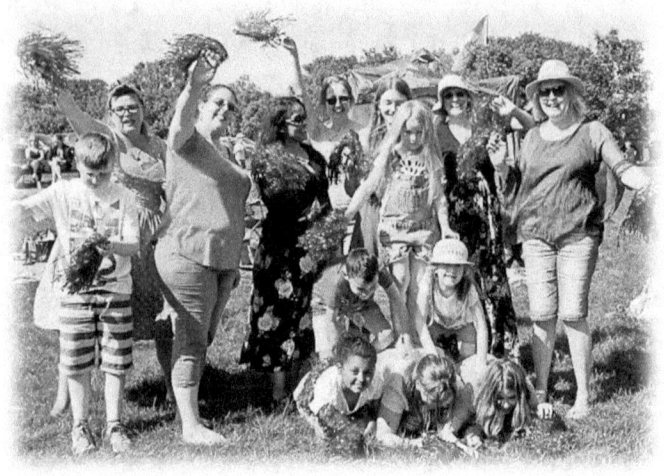

Chapter 7 – Holidays

A CHRISTMAS BLESSING

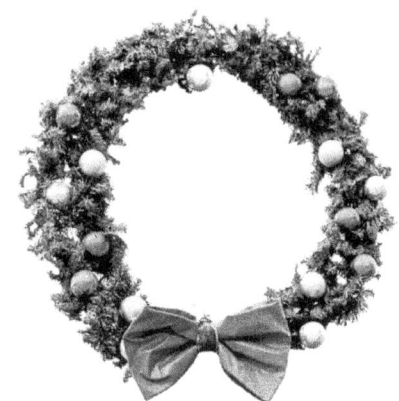

In this season of tinsel, sparkle, and
bright lights,
may you experience the relaxed
confidence that comes with
knowing a light will illuminate your
path every day of the year.

In this season of watching children
enjoy the magic of December,
may you also experience the mystery of Christmas with childlike
anticipation, playfulness, and light hearted fun.

In this season of expectations,
may you hold the present moment with reverence and be at peace with
however future moments evolve.

In this season of remembering Christmas past,
May your ponderings bring you the gifts of comfort, understanding,
healing, and hope.

In this season of gift giving,
may you be blessed with loving relationships, the opportunity to receive,
and the pleasure of spreading kindness. May you know that within
everything that happens there is a precious gift meant just for you.

In this season of gathering together with friends and family,
may you be nourished by the sharing of food, hugs, and an appreciation
of each person's uniqueness. May the support and companionship of
loved ones inspire you. And may you be a good friend to yourself.

In this season that celebrates the guiding star,
may you clearly see the path that leads home to the light and beauty of
the inner Spirit. May nothing ever come between the light and yourself.

In this season of angels singing and people caroling,
may notes of hope, comfort, and gratitude fill your days. May there be
harmony between your inner and outer self, and may the melody of your
soul be present in all you do.

In this season of manger gentleness,
may you remember the tender presence of your infant self as you stood
on the threshold of your life. May you embrace your adult self in an
honoring of the sacredness of your life's journey.

In this season of celebrating the miracle of birth,
may you birth, in the stillness of your soul, an openness to change and
the miracle of grace and growth.

In this season of new beginnings,
may you appreciate the many ways life gives you to start over again –
from the dawning of each new day to the ending of life as we know it,
which is just another beginning.

In this season of seeing with new eyes,
may you celebrate the many forms of love – even those that present
themselves as loss or grief. May you be comforted, and loss and grief
transformed, so you never miss the meaning of an experience.

In this season of peace making,
may you honor all that has been, is now, and will be.

In this season of commemorating where you are right now, this
December 25th,

may you be filled with gratitude for the ongoing gift of your personal journey. May the comforting presence of lessons learned keep you company, and may you know without a doubt that you are never alone.

In this season of gratitude,
may you know that the love that created the first Christmas Day never ends. May you feel its presence - it is here, today, right now, in each one of us.

FINDING OUR NORTH STAR

Stars are often part of Christmas decorations and celebrations. Personally, I love stars all year round, so here are a few thoughts concerning one star that often dominates the sky. For thousands of years the North Star has been a bright guiding light that helped people on their journeys. Our life is also a journey, and we all have an individual North Star within us that guides us to live by our deeply held beliefs and guiding principles. It can be thought of as an internal compass that is unique to each of us, and represents who we are at our deepest level. It represents what is most important to us. It is the compass of the soul that determines the richness of our life.

This doesn't mean we don't ever get lost. Getting lost can be beneficial because, as we work our way through times that feel dark, when choices are difficult or grief is fresh, if we are willing, we will discover treasure. The treasure we carry from our struggles and hardships holds not only value to us, but value to others when we share them as a gift. As C. G. Jung wrote, "One does not become enlightened by imagining figures of light, but by making the darkness conscious."[1]

Everyone's journey is different because our origin and destination are not the same. Because of its history as a navigational tool, the North Star has also become a symbol for personal growth. It's the inner compass that keeps us on course because it knows our passions and purpose. Finding our North Star means we know where we're headed, which creates confidence and resilience. As long as our North Star is wholesome and vital, we can trust the process. It will energize us to stay true to our destination.

There are some clues that tell us when we're out of touch with our North Star. No matter how goal orientated we may appear, if we're feeling a lack of purpose or meaning, we're out of touch. If days feel more like drudgery and we lack enthusiasm, we've lost our connection with our North Star. If we are living our lives according to other people's expectations, we've lost our North Star. Feeling empty, disconnected from our emotions, and hollow inside, is another clue to being out of touch. So, how do we reconnect with our North Star?

Here are a few suggestions for finding our North Star. It can begin with taking responsibility for our own development, which starts with an honest look inside our hearts for our deepest longings. It's time to honor those longings. Then eliminate that inner judgmental voice that tells us we are not good enough – that's just not true. Quiet contemplative time helps bring clarity as we get in touch with our deepest longings. Asking for guidance and journaling afterward can be very effective. Spiritual practices help us find the sacredness in being part of something greater then ourself.

We know deep in our bones what is right for us, so we follow the inner nudges that might indicate a needed change. Since we can't give 100% of ourself to every area of our life, we can choose what is most important to do now with our present circumstances. Remember, as our life changes our priorities are likely to change, too. Playing is important because it helps our creativity and problem-solving abilities. Martha Beck, Ph.D. wrote, "Putting joyful activities into every nook and cranny of your day is a great way to start toward your North Star."[2] Each morning, when we wake up, we can recommit to following our guiding light. Reaching out to people we trust is also important because we all need a strong support system.

Martha Beck wrote, "Identifying your North Star is a deep psychological and spiritual art."[3] It's our guiding principles – something we aim to keep in line with every day. It's what keeps us energized and enthusiastic, making us want to jump out of bed in the morning. It's our direction to the destination of what is most important for our wellbeing. When we are truly authentic, we are living by our North star because it symbolizes the light we can always turn to. It will always be there – it will not let us down. It's the guiding light for our soul's journey. Once we've discovered our North Star, all the other constellations line up. These represent the values and creativity that are guiding our choices. Author David Whyte wrote, "Our genius is to understand, and stand beneath the set of stars present at our birth, and from that place to seek the hidden, single star, over the night horizon, we did not know we were following."[4]

CHANGING THE PRESENT – GIVING DIFFERENTLY

Slowing down and savoring the present moment is a challenge in December. Intentionally a decision was made with our loved ones to encourage a needed change in gift giving, which moved the focus from extensive shopping, to inexpensive but meaningful personalized gifts. This is what I would like to share with you – a look at giving differently.

201

In December a list is circulated offering ideas for giving. When we gather on Christmas day, we have made our selection and come prepared to participate. It is such a meaningful exchange that we move from laughing, to crying, to laughing again, throughout the morning. The following is a list to choose from that symbolizes the 12 days of Christmas.

①Share a favorite quote, poem, short prose, or in your own words, something that encouraged, uplifted, or inspired you.

②Make a list of two or three funny memories you share with at least one person in the room and be ready to tell all.

③Try a handmade gift from the kitchen such as: hot cocoa kit, microwave rice heat bag for neck or back, scented bath salts, or favorite cookie mix kit.

④Choose five or six words that describe a person in the room (or somewhere else) and share why you chose those particular words (keeping it positive – this is Christmas morning).

⑤Tell a truly embarrassing story that you have not told anyone before (maybe just one other person) that would be fun to share.

⑥Share a song that may be sung, played on an instrument, or recorded, with lyrics you enjoy.

⑦Make a coupon book offering your services in any way that would be meaningful to the receiver such as a back and neck massage, dinner, babysitting, painting a room, computer tech support, or a household cleaning project done without complaint.

⑧Create a collage of pictures, inspirational sayings, or recipes that would be meaningful to the receiver.

⑨Put together a snack basket for your football enthusiast.

⑩Gather old jewelry, hats, wigs and clothes to create a dress-up box for children.

⑪Choose to share the memory of one of your favorite tangible or intangible Christmas gifts.

⑫Share with all what you most appreciate in your life right now.

If we take a deep breath, step back, and refocus, we'll discover the joy of simplifying and savoring the Christmas holidays. May this month of December be a time of relaxed enjoyment.

"HAPPINESS HANGOVER"

Christmas and New Year are the biggest holidays of the year so, when they are over, some of us breath a deep sigh of relief, while others feel a disappointing let down. In her book "**A Happy You: Your Ultimate Prescription for Happiness**" Elizabeth Lombardo Ph.D. calls this feeling of post-holiday blues "happiness hangover."[5]

It can happen at the end of any positive event that involves planning and stimulates excitement, so Christmas and New Year are only two possibilities. It can happen after a big wedding, a long-anticipated vacation, a carefully planned family reunion, a graduation, completing a major project, or reaching a health treatment goal. Dr. Lombardo suggests that this can occur any time we focus our energy (physical, emotional, mental, and spiritual) in planning the details, and doing the work involved in creating a significant event.

We thrive on working towards a goal at home, at work, with friends, or with health professionals. We love to share fun and meaningful activities because it's satisfying and rewarding. But, after all that organizing and anticipation, when it's over we can feel let down.

How do we know we have a happiness hangover? We're exhausted so energy is low, we feel down in the dumps, we feel a loss of purpose and wonder "what do I do now?" If we find ourselves with these symptoms Dr. Lombardo has some easy suggestions. First, she suggests gratitude because it shifts our energy from focusing on what is missing, to the appreciation of the people and events we have just experienced. Let's remind ourselves of times in the past when we lost something before we fully knew its value. And let's also remember not to let big events overshadow all the little daily pleasures there are to enjoy.

Her second suggestion is to relive the event through treasured memories. Remember the spontaneous hug from a child, or the laughter during a holiday meal. In our minds we can relive our vacation by recalling the beach sunrise and again feel the warm sand on our bare feet. Going through a picture album slowly savoring every page is delightful, as is watching a video of an event. Put on the T-shirt and listen to the music of that concert you waited so long to attend.

Her third suggestion is to create a new focus. This does not mean we need to immediately jump into another major project – what we need is some recovery time. And in our recovery time we can create something to look forward to while we nourish ourselves. Nature is nourishing so visiting a botanical garden, walking the beach, and sitting in the shade of a tree listening to the wild life all around us is refreshing. If we can't be outside, we can still enjoy nature by watching cloud patterns, or wind playing with the trees while we mentally relive our favorite place to walk. Scheduling a spa day or a massage renews energy, as does quiet reading time in a favorite chair, listening to music, or taking an afternoon nap. As we take care of ourselves, and create a new focus, our energies return.

Happiness hangover disappears quickly when we intentionally choose what brings us pleasure, and treat ourselves with kindness. As we begin a new year, let's give ourselves a large dose of TLC along with gratitude for this past holiday season, this day, this right now moment. There is so much to enjoy and look forward to!

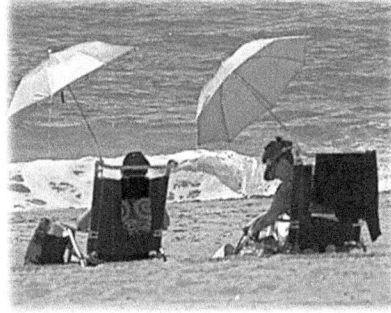

TAKE IT EASY ON YOURSELF

Not realizing how divided my attention was, I headed to my local grocery store for Thanksgiving week shopping. It was three days before Thanksgiving. I arrived at 8:20am. Walking into the store I realized I had forgotten to bring my latest collection of recyclable bags to put in the bin outside the store's front door. A few minutes later I realized I had left my reusable bags in the car. And shortly after that I lost my grocery list. Retracing my steps didn't help in locating the lost list so I decided to walk down each isle to stimulate my memory. There were numerous shoppers in the store making progress slow. When finally checking out, I remarked to the cashier that I had come early hoping to avoid a crowd. She replied that I had avoided the crowd, assuring me that in another hour the store would be jammed with three times as many people.

Feeling frazzled, I left the store and started driving home. I was getting ready to say unkind things to myself, and give myself a hard time, when I turned on the radio. The first song to play was "Take It Easy On Yourself" written by Don Williams[6]. It was exactly what I needed to hear. Right then I decided that phrase was my mantra for the holidays. I also decided

I needed to stay in the moment. It's the only way to go through the holidays without forgetting and loosing things because attention is divided.

There was a New York Times article by Jolie Kerr titled "How to Survive the Holidays."[7] She acknowledges the joys and stresses of the holidays and offers some sound advice. Here are a few of her suggestions. Set a Christmas budget and stick to it to eliminate after Christmas regrets. It spoils the fun to be paying for Christmas in July. Put yourself on your gift list. Treat yourself to something that makes you feel good. It's important to give ourselves some TLC.

Jolie suggests focusing on only those extra Christmas activities that mean the most to us, so we don't feel depleted half way through December. Prioritize and say "no" to everything else. When dealing with visitors, we all enjoy those prized friendships don't we? The ones we invite in for a visit without thinking about when the house was last cleaned.

If you have critical friends or relatives, kindly stop any disrespectful remarks. Stop that from entering your sacred living space. Invitations are not issued to toxic people. If this Christmas involves serious health issues you especially need to "take it easy on yourself." Eliminate any guilt about making personal needs a priority. Clearly state your boundaries and insist they be honored. Remember, the people who are objecting to your limits are the ones who are benefiting most from your having none.

Let's let go of mistakes, they are part of our learning process. Rather than focus on what we can't change, let's refocus on what we can change and give it our best. Let's celebrate our own uniqueness instead of comparing ourselves to other people. And if we find ourselves cranky, let's take a look at the kind of pressure we're putting on ourselves. Of all the months of the year, December is the one where we need to be most kind to ourselves. The best part of Christmas falls into what Fred Rogers said,

"That which is essential is invisible to the naked eye."[8] What is essential is our "well of inner love" that leads to all our expressions of love. What is essential is knowing in our soul that all is well. What is essential is viewing the world through a lens of kindness toward our diversity. These are the things that touch us deeply. It is essential to "take it easy on ourselves" this December and enjoy what's most important to each of us.

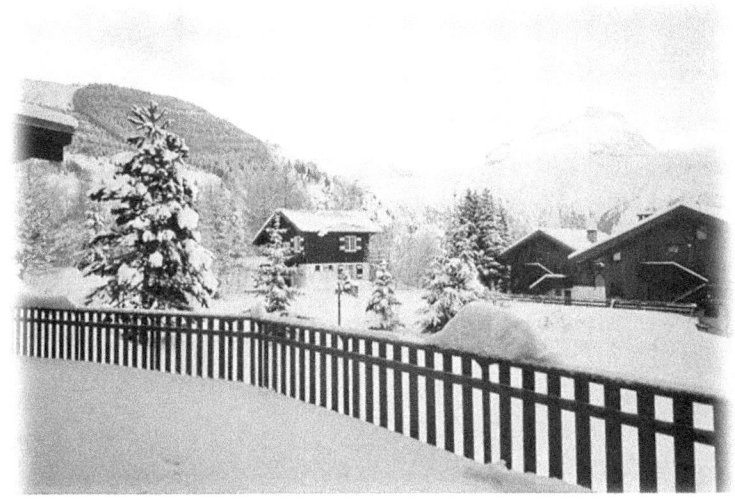

Chapter 8 – Dealing With Illness

ASKING FOR WHAT WE NEED

"Thank you, I would appreciate some help."

How many times have you heard someone say, "Let me know if you need anything." It can be a difficult offer to accept. Sometimes we feel overwhelmed and don't know how to answer, we worry about being a burden, or we believe asking for help is a sign of weakness. When was the last time you felt comfortable asking anyone for anything? We desire, we want, we need, without asking.

Clearly stating needs and wants is something I'm working on, and I remind myself that hinting is not the same as asking. The family I grew up in did not model clarity in asking for help, advice, directions, or information, so that skill did not come with me into adulthood. It was frustrating to experience my hints not turning into the results I desired, until I realized the problem was my lack of clarity. This skill needs practice which is best done starting small and being emotionally calm.

We need to start by clarifying what we need or want. Sometimes we just don't know, so it's hard to ask effectively. If we give ourselves time to think through the changes we need, we will be able to verbalize our needs effectively. We need to get past being dissatisfied and take time to create a detailed picture of what we do want. Complaining, whining, or hinting is not the same as describing the outcome we need. We need to be clear and direct in sharing our description for change.

We are not at our best if we are being irrational or emotional so, for maximum success, we need to restore calmness before negotiating needed help. Sometimes wishful thinking is a place where we can get stuck. It produces no change and leaves us feeling denied the help we thought was coming. If we choose not to ask, and stay in wishful thinking, we create a constant state of deprivation for ourselves. Who needs that!

So, let's get specific about both big issues and small. Ask the kids to pick up their toys. Ask when the next sale will be (one of my favorite requests). Ask the name of a paint color and then ask where you can find it. See a great hair cut? Ask who did it and where to go. Ask for a raise or a deadline extension. Ask for help with meal preparation, laundry, or house cleaning. Paperwork pilling up? Ask for help organizing (something I love to do). Ask for a personal hour just for yourself to reclaim inner peacefulness. Just be clear about what it is you need.

For those of us dealing with any major health issue, the needs can be numerous. To make medical appointments most effective, ask for a driver and a companion who can take notes on what the doctor is saying. If needed, ask for a second doctor's opinion. Ask what your treatment choices are, and insist on respect for your individual journey. Inquire what support groups are available. Ask for respect from all caregivers.

When aid is offered let's reply with, "Thank you, I would appreciate some help." Responding with a grateful heart will boost our immune system and could be the beginning or the strengthening of a friendship. Occasional disappointments will happen, but they can be handled with flexibility. I think we'll be surprised by how many people come through for us when we ask for what we need. Just ask.

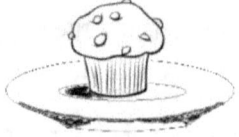

CELEBRATIONS AREN'T JUST FOR HOLIDAYS

We generally take time to celebrate life's big events like weddings, birthdays, graduations, and holidays. Of course, these are important, but what if we broadened our perspective and gave ourselves permission to celebrate life's little things? Life is full of little events, so starting a celebration would depend on our creativity. When we appreciate the little things in life, our focus is directed towards what is fun, nurturing, and uplifting, instead of what is irritating, frustrating, or hurtful. This means practicing gratitude for the everyday things we often take for granted, or miss altogether. This doesn't mean negative events will disappear, but it will keep us from over-emphasizing their significance in our lives.

If we slow down and savor our days, we will discover all kinds of things to celebrate. How about bringing out the champagne when we remember to laugh and not take ourselves so seriously. Have a celebrative cup of coffee with a friend because it's Tuesday. Sleeping in could be celebratory after a series of early morning risings. Completing another session of chemo or radiation is worth a splurge of self-pampering. Celebrate the beautiful gift of encouragement from a friend, or enjoy a beach walk after several rainy days in a row. This morning my husband and I celebrated the omelet he made that was only lightly browned on the outside and moist inside. We chose not to dwell on omelets of the past which were a bit scary. I like to celebrate completing household cleaning tasks with time in my favorite recliner chair reading my current library book.

Being diagnosed with cancer doesn't mean there's nothing left to celebrate. For Ivanna Kern[1], having appendix cancer led her into appreciating every day, and celebrating the host of little things that make up our lives. With enthusiasm, her friends and family eagerly joined in the fun. She recently celebrated what she calls her "sixth cancerversary." Looking at everyday as a gift, she had a series of "chemo parties" marking the time she was half way through her treatment schedule, then done with treatment, and finally cancer free.

She described her uplifted spirit when she received a prayer shawl from people she didn't know. Then someone gave her a stone to keep in her pocket with the encouraging message to "Be Strong." The laughter of every gathering of her support group, combined with the pleasure of being silly, filled her with positive emotions and energized her for whatever came next. Now, cancer free, she continues to celebrate and embrace life by paying attention to daily details with deep gratitude.

These kinds of celebrations create positive emotions which boost our immune systems, and allow us to recover more quickly from physical illness. Even if recovery isn't possible, we still become psychologically resilient and are able to be more creative and flexible. That sounds remarkably helpful, because when the tough stuff comes, it's positive emotions that will help us balance and cope. Learning how to appreciate and celebrate the little things in life is a powerful tool for physical and mental health. Today, I'm celebrating sister time with a lunch just for the two of us - what are you celebrating?

COLOR'S GIFTS

After a tiring thirteen-hour plane ride to Singapore, I gratefully exited the plane and wearily walked into the airport, hoping it wouldn't take too long to find my luggage and hotel. After the dull colors in the airplane, I was delighted to see large containers of blooming flowers and small trees down every walking isle, all the way from the disembarking area to the exit door of the terminal. In the background soft classical music was playing as I eagerly feasted on all the colors of the blossoms and leaves in front of me. I gradually felt my energy renewing. It was so nourishing that I went from weary walking to having a spring in my step, and from worrying about how to make all my connections, to relaxing into the process. The airport planners were using color psychology to destress tired travelers and it sure worked for me.

Everyday we're surrounded by a glorious array of colors that are influencing us, whether we are aware of it or not. Colors create mood, convey information, trigger physical reactions, and even influence what we purchase. Color psychology is a growing field of study that I find fascinating. Why do we feel so good when we're walking through autumn's beautifully colored trees? Think of the colors we use in expressions that describe emotions like; "I'm green with envy," or "They're so angry they see red," or "I'm feeling down and blue." Jazz even plays the "blues." Our feelings about colors are both personal and cultural. For example, Western countries view white as representing purity and freshness, but in Eastern countries it is a symbol of mourning.

In our local publication of 32963, the February 13, 2020 edition featured an article by Caroline Leaper titled, "Why wearing color is proven to have good mental benefits."[2] It talked about all the bright colors worn on the 2020 red carpet, and how color affects both the wearer and the viewer. In the article there is this quote by Jules Standish, "Our reaction to seeing inspiring, bright, harmonious things is mood lifting, which in turn has a physical effect, improving blood pressure and strengthening the nervous system."[3] We impact ourselves and the people around us because colors that stimulate create a neurological response.

Standish also says, "Every color has a purpose, an influence and a power to change the way we look and feel about ourselves and the way others view us too." On the color spectrum there are warm colors and cool colors. The warm colors of red, orange, and yellow can speed up our metabolism and evoke emotions ranging from warmth, comfort, and satisfaction, to feelings of frustration and anger if there's an overdose. Cool colors include blue, purple, and green which promote calmness, serenity and relaxation, as well as sadness and ambivalence if experienced in overwhelming amounts.

Color's gifts are ours for the taking, and those of us with cancer know how important it is to feel good even on our most challenging days. Color psychology works, so wear that brightly colored outfit to your chemo treatment, you'll give yourself and everyone in the room a serotonin lift. Wear your favorite color top and pants on your days at home to keep your spirits up. Have some bright scarfs and caps handy to make you smile while encouraging your hair to regrow. Wear your warm power colors to each doctor visit to remind yourself that you are the one making the decisions. Choose a soft afghan in a cool calming color for napping, and give yourself pictures to enjoy in your home that have tranquil colors to encourage peace of mind. Look in your clothes closet, identify what pieces make you feel happy, and wear them with enthusiasm.

We can get out whatever art supplies we have (a box of crayons will do) and show all our inner feelings in every shade and hue we need to relieve stress or express joy. Use color's gifts to keep yourself encouraged, uplifted, creatively expressing who you are with every color of the rainbow. Here's to being our own beautiful, unique, colorful selves.

DEFINING OUR NON-NEGOTIABLES

Defining non-negotiables means identifying and living with what is most important to us. This is a sacred promise we make to ourself that reflects the values and principles we live by. They clearly define what we will or won't accept from others, or ourself, and are a statement on how we want to be treated. These are the items that, if disrespected, are deal breakers. This commitment to our highest priorities will be unique to each of us and our particular circumstances.

Non-negotiables can be thought of as a steady anchor that keeps us from floating through life without a clear sense of direction. Without a steady anchor we can be easily influenced by events and people, loosing ourself, and what we hold dear. When we show up for ourself and each other, honoring our boundaries, we build relationships on respect and trust and we build our own self-confidence.

When we choose our non-negotiables, we need to choose what we have control over. If someone treats us poorly and we stand up for ourself, that person might not like it, but they will know what our boundaries are so we're less likely to be treated that way again. Let's remember we don't have control of the outcome, but we do have control of our boundaries.

The process can start by listing a few top priorities. Stephen Covey writes, "You have to decide what your highest priorities are and have the courage – pleasantly, smilingly, non-apologetically, to say "no" to other things. And the way you do that is by having a bigger "yes" burning inside. The enemy of the "best" is often the "good"."[4]

The yes is our non-negotiable which could be: respectful relationships, being kind to ourself when we make mistakes, taking Sunday off from electronics, family time, or daily spiritual practices. Our list reflects the core things that sustain us. I read a story of a woman who loved to give dinner parties. She held everyone responsible for the attitude and behavior they brought into her home, so when a guest made a disrespectful remark, they were ushered out the front door and never invited in again. They violated her boundary of respectful behavior.

A change in circumstances may add new non-negotiables to the list. When I had cancer, I went through 6 surgeries in ten months. Life felt like I was either recovering from surgery, or getting ready for another one.

Two new non-negotiables for me were small meals, and few visitors, so I could have the quiet healing time required. This was again an issue of respect. Anyone going through chemo or radiation needs to set some ground rules, because even well-intentioned friends and family can be overwhelming.

A present boundary for me is closing the door and insisting that no one disturb me when I am writing. I need my concentration unbroken, so I am practicing my commitment to self-care. I also honor my husband's need not to be disturbed when he is painting. Non-negotiables are not luxuries, but are the anchor which supports everything else. They aren't saved for emergencies, but are a part of everyday life.

Communicating our non-negotiables to the people in our life who mean the most enables them to support us, and keeps us accountable. This takes us to our highest level of integrity. When we become our own best friend, we only allow people into our sacred space who value who we are, and are important to our well-being.

Since our top priorities are the anchor for everything else, let's take time to identify them. We'll be happier, more productive, and experience richer relationships as a result. We can all experience the deep satisfaction of defining and living by our non-negotiables, which will enhance every day of our life.

EMBRACING THE ORDINARY

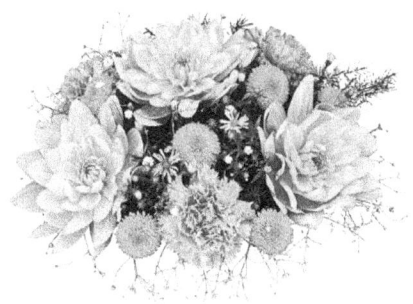

We are the curators of our own
contentment, but sometimes we
don't appreciate the contentment
we find in the ordinary until we are
faced with something unexpected,
difficult or challenging. It can be anything from a close call in a car (my
husband) or airplane, financial struggles, a career change or a serious
illness (me). It's anything that wakes us up to the pleasure and wonder of
ordinary days.

Being diagnosed with breast cancer opened my eyes to the delight
possible in the details of a day, especially during the times when I could
not take care of myself. I slowly had to work my way back to
independence, and along the way I learned some valuable lessons. There
was a lot of recovery time needed with multiple surgeries which meant
more than the usual time at home. Necessity gave me the gift of slowness
which heightened my awareness of everything going on around me. And
I celebrated every little bit of independence that each day brought, even
if it was only going to the bathroom by myself (ordinary yes, but a big
deal after surgery because that function was taken for granted). Other
functions had been taken for granted as well.

The ordinary daily sounds and activities had always been present, but
now I was in a spirit of gratitude, paying close attention. There was
pleasure in hearing the tea kettle whistle, seeing the brilliant colors of
fruits and vegetables being chopped in the kitchen, the fragrance of
homemade soup, the rustle of book pages while reading in bed, the
texture of a soft afghan, a glass of cold water on my night table, gentle
music in the background, the hum of the washing machine taking care of
the laundry. Rick Field says, "When we pay attention, whatever we're

doing – whether it be cooking, cleaning or making love – is transformed......We begin to notice details and textures that we never noticed before; everyday life becomes clearer, sharper, and at the same time more spacious."[5] From this perspective little things begin to mean a lot and we engage more deeply with the present moment.

Mary Jean Irion invites us to revel in the ordinary with this thought. "Normal day, let me be aware of the treasure you are. Let me learn from you, love you, bless you before you depart. Let me not pass you by in quest of some rare and perfect tomorrow. Let me hold you while I may, for it may not always be so. One day I shall dig my nails into the earth, or bury my face into a pillow, or stretch myself taught, or raise my hands to the sky and want, more than all the world, your return."[6]

The idea is to appreciate and embrace the ordinary without having a crisis, so living in awareness becomes the norm. I don't want to be sick in order to be observant. Today let's identify more of those joyful simplicities that offer a deep sense of personal comfort, because our sense of well-being is the highest priority. No matter where we are in our healing journey, discovering our own small delights will bring us peace and pleasure, and who of us can't use a little more of that! Let's embrace the ordinary together.

HOLDING HANDS

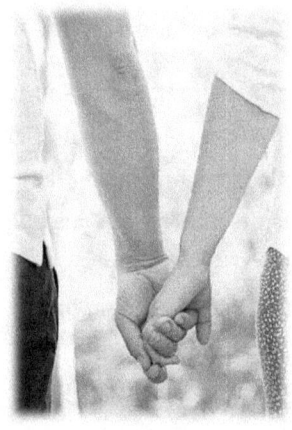

During the medical test I was told not to move except for breathing. A long needle was inserted into my breast, pulled partially out, repositioned, and inserted deeply again a number of times. This process was painful. It also lasted longer than I expected. All I could think about was being perfectly still so this test did not need to be repeated! Finally, I reached the point of no longer being able to contain my tears and they quietly slid down my face. A nurse standing beside me slipped her hand under the blanket covering me, and held my hand. That changed everything!

I was no longer alone. I immediately knew someone in the room understood how difficult this was, and was giving me an active sign of support. Her personal attention acknowledged both my physical and emotional needs, and formed a bond of solidarity between us. While my tears ran unchecked, she gave me eye contact, told me where we were in the process, and held my hand until the test was finished. She gave me the gift of being completely present, and her physical touch reassured me of her focused attention and caring concern.

When I look back on that test I remember that the pain was balanced by the kindness of a stranger. I don't even know her name but I remember what she did for me. Her thoughtfulness made all the difference. She used the simple act of holding hands to communicate personal support in a cold, sterile room where everyone else was focused on the process, not the person.

It was a gift given with perfect timing, and a reminder of how important small gestures can be. The difficulty of my test was quietly acknowledged, and her gentle act of holding my hand confirmed that I was seen and understood. "Holding hands is a promise to one another that, just for the moment, the two of you don't have to face the whole world alone." (unknown author) Holding hands has taken on a whole new meaning for me.

When we are truly present for the people around us we listen with eye contact, and become mindful, attentive, and aware. Putting down our phones and stepping away from our computers is the doorway into the shared comfort of the holding hands experiences. We open ourselves up to more intimate opportunities when we affirm our support for anyone going through a difficult time. Emily Kimbrough writes, "Remember, we all stumble, every one of us. That's why it's a comfort to go hand in hand."[7]

This is what happens in support groups – we walk hand in hand. Along with that we also hug, listen, laugh, and respect changing needs. We honor the importance of time alone to process what is happening. The comfort and security of holding hands makes whatever is happening a bit easier. Let's enjoy being truly present with each other, and share the simple, priceless treasure found in the meaningful connection of holding hands.

KEEPING A GRATITUDE JOURNAL

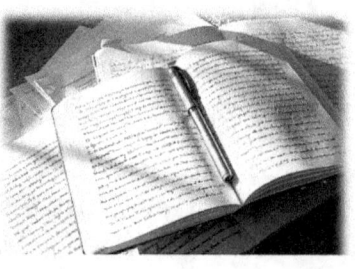

Today my journals from various times in my life came out for a review. For three years my husband and I lived in England and, because it was such a unique experience, I journaled our various adventures of learning to live in another culture. It was scary, challenging, priority-changing, and loads of fun. While rereading some of my English journals I was grateful for all the writing I did, recording details that memory alone can forget over time. As I read, I was easily reminded of the personal growth that comes when everything familiar is left behind. Right in front of me was the value of lessons learned that I don't want to forget. Journaling keeps it all alive.

And then out came my gratitude journals. Perusing through the year 2014 (my year with cancer) again revealed how therapeutic keeping a gratitude journal can be; not only at the time of writing, but also to look back and see again all the little daily miracles that were present. Even during the hardest days, I could see how people were reaching out to me, loving me, and encouraging me through the whole process of multiple surgeries until I was finally cancer-free.

During that time my goal was to write in my journal three things I was thankful for at the end of each day. I discovered it was hard to stop at three (so I didn't) because there were so many more! Doing this before bed filled my mind with appreciation for the gifts of the day, and also created a positive focus to take to sleep with me. This helped even the toughest days feel better because my focus was on the amazing ways love carried me through that challenging experience.

Journals don't need to be fancy books with leather covers – any notebook works well. And entries don't need to be long to be meaningful. The treasure is in what we choose to write in them. A crisis usually brings us to a crossroads where choices invite new beginnings. Expressing our gratitude keeps its positive energy active, and creates an ever-increasing spiral of appreciation. Brother David Steindl-Rast sums it up this way: "As I express my gratitude, I become more deeply aware of it. And the greater my awareness, the greater my need to express it. What happens here is a spiraling ascent, a process of growth in ever-expanding circles around a steady center."[8] Looking back on what we journal is a window through which we see how blessed we are, how well we were cared for, and how the same loving, supportive care is ours today and every day.

Melody Beattie said it beautifully in this quote: "Gratitude unlocks the fullness of life. It turns what we have into enough, and more. It turns denial into acceptance, chaos to order, confusion to clarity. It can turn a meal into a feast, a house into a home, or a stranger into a friend. Gratitude makes sense of our past, brings peace for today, and creates a vision for tomorrow."[9] Journaling gratitude is a gift to ourself and anyone we care to share it with. May your day be filled with miracles large and small to record in your own private journal.

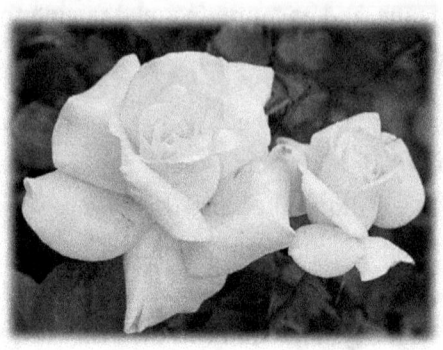

LIVING IN-BETWEEN

Sometimes in life we have to let go of what is familiar, without fully knowing what will come next, and live in an in-between place. It's that time when we are moving from where we are now to where we want to be. It can be in-between jobs, homes, relationships, goals, behaviors, feelings or health issues, and it's hard to leave what's familiar and step into the unknown. This isn't fun, but it is necessary for our health on all levels. We might even feel like we are standing still, but we're not – we're in the in-between place and still moving forward.

This came home to me when I was diagnosed with ductal carcinoma breast cancer, and I knew my life would never be the same. It was time for me to let go of what was familiar and embrace the unknown, (easier said than done) which brought a steady flow of change in the form of in-between experiences. I chose to have a double mastectomy and reconstruction so, first there was three weeks in-between my diagnosis and my first surgery, when I wondered if something more would be discovered during the operation. That was followed with time in-between five further surgeries, healing time between each surgery, and learning how to take care of my new breasts (we're good friends now). It's hard to prepare for the unknown and unsettling to live with it.

Living in-between usually stirs up our emotions and among the first to arrive are fear, apprehension, and anxiety. As soon as I was given my cancer diagnosis, I went right into fear. I asked my Higher Power for something to hang onto and immediately came across the following quote from Parker Palmer, "I will always have fears, but I need not be my fears, for I have other places within myself from which to speak and act."[10] That became a well-used mantra. Then I read this written by Mark Nepo, "More than anything, fear blinds, and only by stepping without hesitation into the next inch of the unknown can we build confidence in the life we are about to live."[11] In working through our emotions, we may feel like we're falling apart, but it is in the falling apart that we are put back together again with new insights, wisdom, and clarity.

Letting go of the illusion of control goes with being in-between. We can't alter the timing of what is happening, or rush the process we are in. Trying to force change to happen quickly is just as ineffective and destructive as change that comes too late. Wisdom, knowledge, and clarity can't be forced. We can't gain perspective before the time is right. How our present circumstances will work into the larger scheme of life is not yet clear. Melody Beattie writes, "We can let go of our need to figure things out, to feel in control. Now is the time to be. To feel. To go through it. To allow things to happen. To learn. To let whatever is being worked out in us take its course. In hindsight we will know. Perspective will come in retrospect."[12]

Life is cyclical and, if we're open to what each cycle brings, we can make the most of each time we enter living in-between. If we are willing to dedicate our time to birth, then we can trust the process we are in. By trusting the process, we become like a flower ready to blossom. Mark

Nepo writes this, "For the flower, it is fully open at each step of its blossoming. The simple rose, at each moment of its slow blossoming, is as open as it can be. The same is true of our lives. In each stage of our unfolding, we are stretched as much as possible. For the human heart is quite slow to blossom."[13] Nature takes time and patience, but if we're willing to let it unfold naturally, its full beauty can be seen. And, if we are patient with our own transformation, we will also see its full beauty. Living in-between is a gifted time offering us more than we can imagine. Things will work out – all is well.

"NOT YET"

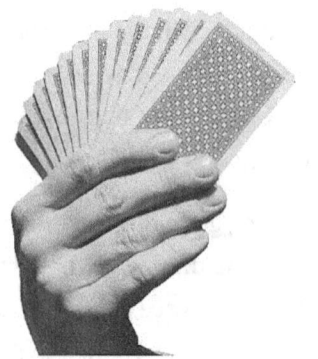

In a TEDx talk, Dr. Carol Dweck of Stanford University described a high school in Chicago that does not give a failing grade when a student doesn't pass a class. Instead, they give a "**Not Yet**". In Dr. Dweck's words, "This shift from outcome to process implies eventual success, and in the meantime, focuses on effort, strategy, resilience, and perseverance. Believing you can improve, instead of assuming you're stuck with the cards you were dealt, makes all the difference."[14]

What an insightful way to encourage ongoing effort. Shifting from outcome to process is helpful when we think of taking a trip. When it comes to traveling, some people want to get there as quickly as possible and look at arrival as the goal (outcome). Other people experience traveling beginning the minute they leave home (process). When the focus is on arriving, adventures along the way such as new people to talk to, ethnic food to try, or beautiful scenery are missed. When we savor every moment, the whole experience is one of pleasure and relaxation, which is what we want a trip to be all about. As T.S. Elliot wrote, "The journey, not the arrival matters."[15]

There are many "Not Yet" moments in our journey through life that lead to reaching for our potential, and valuing the process. Those of us who have dealt with cancer, or any major illness, know there are markers along the way that say we're in process, but not there yet. The doctor visits, surgeries, treatment plans, waiting for test results, and specialist referrals are all part of the journey. Along the way we meet new people that often become dear friends; we see places we wouldn't ordinarily see, and try new therapies. We hear inspirational stories that lift our spirits, and we find humor in the most unexpected places.

This is using the effort, strategy, resilience, and perseverance Dr. Dweck mentions. We deepen our understanding of ourselves, clarify our goals, and know that even though we're still "Not Yet" where we want to be, we're on our way. In between the tough stuff are times of fun and play that keep us going. It's never too late to finish something we started long ago or to begin something new.

Life is more enjoyable if we take in the scenery along the way, enjoy new experiences, and meet those people who are friends in the making. As Dr. Dweck suggests, when we focus on effort, strategy, perseverance, and resilience we can turn that "Not Yet" into the beginning of the next chapter in our journey. No matter what stage of the journey we're in, the process is always with us. It's the devotion, dedication, and hard work that make each of us a success story. In Serena Williams words, "A champion is defined not by their wins, but by how they recover when they fall."[16]

STEPPING BACK, MOVING FORWARD

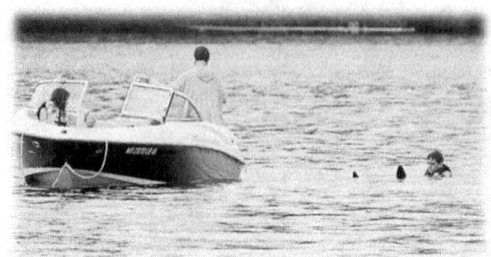

Remember the movie, *Back to the Future?* Yes, that one; where going back can impact future outcome. A recent ocean beach walk through newly deposited seaweed reminded me of this truth.

My childhood summers were spent on a lake in Wisconsin. My parents trusted my brother and I to responsibly handle their water ski boat (it was too much fun to lose that privilege by doing something stupid) and there was nothing we enjoyed more than a day of lake activities. When friends came over it felt like life couldn't get any better.

Driving the boat, we skimmed over the water loving the wind in our hair while we checked out all the other activities on the lake. There were a few places to avoid like the large rock that was mostly submerged, and the resort that had lots of seaweed floating on top of the water in front of it.

But there was another obstacle that wasn't easily seen. Each summer there was a period of time when a certain kind of seaweed grew from the bottom of the lake to about five inches beneath the surface of the water. During our boating activities this seaweed could wrap itself around the boat's propeller and build up until the engine bogged down and alerted us to stop and "clean prop".

The best way to get free of the seaweed was to put the engine in reverse. The seaweed would quickly unwind and float to the top of the water. But before we went forward again, we would hand check (with the engine in neutral – another area not to be stupid) and remove any remaining seaweed. Without removing the seaweed, the engine would overheat and break down, so there was no going forward again without going backward first. We respectfully gave that engine everything it needed to keep going forward.

Right there, surrounded by beach seaweed, I had an aha moment. I began to think of the times in my life when I needed to step back to release the seaweed of events, attitudes, or judgements from others or myself before I could move forward again. Then I realized life repeatedly offers us that opportunity. Giving up things that weigh us down is one way to back up and then move forward.

Letting other people's opinions control our decision making is something that can weigh us down (seaweed in the prop). This is especially true if we are making decisions about our health. We can listen to what other people think, but the decisions are ours. When we're dealing with cancer, or any major illness, we choose the doctors, the treatment plan, the drugs we are willing to take and those we are not. And if we need to redo our treatment plan, we step back, make needed changes and move forward again.

Let's take a step back and release our past from weighing us down (clean the prop). There is no shame in making mistakes – it's how we learn. Anthony Gucciardi writes, "The butterfly does not look back at the caterpillar in shame, just as you should not look back on your past in shame. Your past was part of your transformation."[17] Let's gather up that hard earned wisdom from the past, and bring it forward to this moment so we can make the changes needed to go forward.

Life can catch us by surprise like the unseen seaweed growing just beneath the water's surface. We may stop but we don't need to get stuck. Whatever our challenges are, if we take a moment to step back and gain perspective, we can move forward with confidence and courage.

THE CLOSET THAT WENT BERZERK!

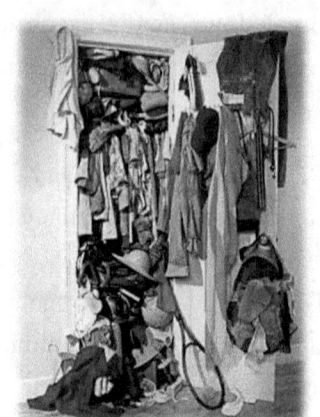

You may have one of these in your house. It's that area that used to be completely organized, or at least passably organized, that suddenly takes on the persona of something that is both scary and out of control. No longer can anything be found because the area has gone berserk.

Recently a closet in my house did that and I was taken by surprise. Every other closet is organized and easy to work in, what happened to this one? All I could do was stand in the middle of the storage room, shaking my head, and slowly begin to acknowledge the numerous times both my husband and I had hurriedly shoved items anywhere, to be put in their proper place later. Later never came.

There were hints of trouble along the way but they were ignored. I was living the Ellen DeGeneres philosophy of, "Procrastinate now, don't put it off."[18] When I was finally willing to look at it the mess was overwhelming.

When working with anything gone berserk, the only way to keep sanity is to divide the project into very small tasks, and do a little each day. Ignoring the rest of the mess, I began on my project shelves sorting what to keep, recycle, or donate. Once that was completed, I experienced such a strong feeling of accomplishment that I could begin looking at other shelves. This new project is ongoing, but at least one box is addressed each day, and I am lighter in mind and spirit as clutter is sorted and reduced. Outer order brings inner calm.

Ignoring a mess only makes it worse, not just in our homes but in our health as well. My mother ignored all the signs of ill health in her body.

When she was told she had cancer, it was so far advanced that she died a month after her diagnosis. She showed me what happens when we don't pay attention to our bodies and, like clutter, let symptoms accumulate. My sister and I have both had cancer only it was diagnosed early and our outcomes were entirely different from Mother.

If we don't take care of ourselves, our health can become unmanageable. Nothing is too small to mention to our doctors, and nothing is insignificant when we are dealing with a serious illness. The treatment process can be overwhelming, but if we take one day, or one hour, or one minute at a time it's manageable. Let's affirm to ourselves and each other that we have the strength, courage, and ability to face any challenge as it comes. Let's call on resolve and confidence to avoid the disaster of procrastination. And let's claim the inner peace that comes when we're taking our day's one small step at a time.

Our homes affect our physical and mental wellbeing so we need to make them a place of comfort, calm, and restoration. Berserk does not foster health on any level. So, little by little we clear the clutter, the closet, and the calendar. We keep each appointment, show up for each test, follow the treatment plan, and commit to our health and wellbeing. Whether it's a closet or cancer, let's avoid going berserk!

THE GIFT OF TEARS

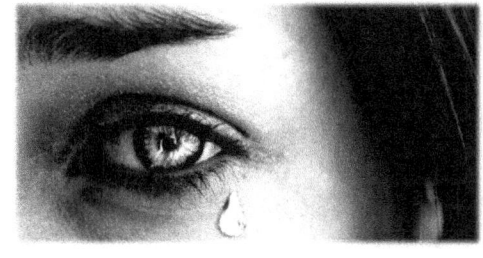

What would we do without the ability to release our emotions when life seems difficult? Let's let those tears roll down our cheeks and not confine ourself to the few tears we think society will allow. I'm suggesting that it's time to embrace the cry that makes our eyes red and our nose run so we're cleansed of built-up emotions. It's the beauty of the safety valve of crying that makes it a gift.

Sometimes tears aren't seen as a gift. Instead, they're seen as something that happens at embarrassingly inconvenient times showing weakness and lack of emotional control. The opposite is true. Eight years ago, when I was grieving the loss of both breasts to cancer in an upcoming surgery, I started crying in the middle of Publix (local grocery store) and couldn't stop. Grabbing a can of tomatoes, I turned my back to the isle and tried to look absorbed in reading the ingredients list (it said tomatoes) while using a lot of Kleenex. Then I decided to raise my head, finish my shopping with no apologies for my wet face, and ignore the strange looks I was getting. Sometimes our emotional releases, essential as they are, do come at inconvenient times. And sometimes we do lose emotional control, but when our mental health just can't wait, we give it the time it needs.

Of course, tears are used to express a variety of emotions. I suspect we've all cried for joy as well as sorrow, but what happens when we repress the feelings that make us cry. Here is some of what I learned from Leo Newhouse[19] who writes for *Harvard Health*. Repressed feelings result in a depressed immune system, heart disease, high blood pressure, increased stress, anxiety and depression. Let's use the gift of tears to avoid that.

Medical studies continue to give us strong evidence that tears are actually healthy and therapeutic. Leo Newhouse also shared some of the benefits of tears. Of course, tears keep our eyes healthy and hydrated, but there's more to it than that. Stress relief happens because tears are composed of stress hormones which get flushed out when we cry, so we naturally detoxify. When toxins are released, we lower our blood pressure and this is why we often feel better after we've had a hard cry. Tears allow us to embrace what's difficult so we can take whatever step is needed next. This can produce a great sense of relief.

Emotional and physical pain is reduced because crying releases oxytocin and endorphins which are feel good hormones. This in turn can improve our sleep. Crying is a powerful tool for our mental health because tears release negativity which results in a rebalanced body. The grieving process needs tears to help move us through its different stages until we get to acceptance, which is the indicator of a healthy recovery.

When we cry, we become vulnerable and real. Because our guard is down, we are more open to connecting with others. Tears break down the barriers we put up with the people around us, as well as ourself. They are the human equalizer that shifts our perspective. Shared tears can be bonding, which benefits our social health and strengthens our relationships as we reach out to each other in mutual support. Crying encourages closeness and empathy. Tears are a basic and unifying experience that is both powerful and important. Let's have the courage to cry without apologies and support each other in this healthy, therapeutic expression. Whatever we're presently processing, accepting this gift enhances our health on all levels.

WHAT'S IN YOUR WELLNESS TOOLKIT?

Toolkits are a part of life – we have one in the trunk of our car, one in the house, and one in my husband's work shop, so when a need arises, we are prepared. Here's a suggestion for another 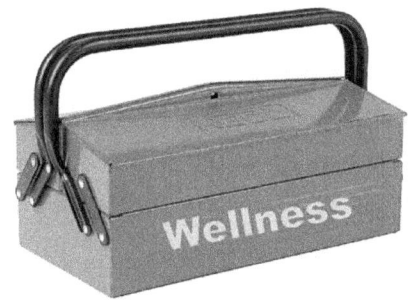 kind of took kit just for wellness. Tools are the habits, products and self-kindness practices that improve the quality of our life. They support us and keep us grounded, anchoring our body, mind and spirit. These are the tools we go to when we want to improve or maintain our wellness and, since we each have our own unique bodies, each person's toolkit will be different and change over time. With the right tools we can improve our well-being any time we want.

To get our ideas flowing it can be helpful to see what other people have in their toolkits. A few of my favorite tools are quiet time, practicing gratitude, deep breathing, spiritual resources (inspirational reading, prayer, meditation) time away from my smartphone, reading historical novels and true stories, kayaking, soup making, time with loved ones, having a good belly laugh, and nature walks. I have one friend that renews herself by cooking up a feast, another makes artistic quilts and another enjoys knitting. When we're stressed in any way, doing something calming is healthy self-care. It helps to make a list of what nourishes us and keep it close by for easy reference. If our tool lists make us feel positive, renewed, and hopeful then we have what we need.

Here are suggestions others have shared. Journaling thoughts, feelings and dreams can be therapeutic. The right kind of music, whether we're listening or making our own, will release tension and restore peace. Another tool is living mindfully which means focusing on the present moment instead of living on autopilot. Taking care of our bodies with good nutrition and appropriate activity belongs in our toolkit. So is being around people who are supportive and make us feel good about ourself. Clothing psychology tells us to wear something that makes us feel good when we need a boost. The tool of spiritual practices often opens us to see new choices and the gifts difficult situations can contain. This is centering and soothing.

Some of us do crossword puzzles or sudoku, play with a pet or rock an infant. Others of us benefit from looking at pictures of people we love who live away from us or focusing on the beauty of a fresh flower. Taking a warm bath or shower is relaxing. More tool suggestions are fishing, gardening, photography, or any hobby that relaxes us. Taking a break from social media is essential for peace of mind so this is worth considering. One tool we all need is getting enough sleep.

When we set our priorities so we're clear about what we can realistically do in one day, and feel compassion for ourself at the end of the day, we're into healthy self-care and have added an important tool to our kit. Our tools help us build resilience, manage stress, build a support system and cope with change. Our toolboxes will be as varied as we are and will change with circumstances, but their usefulness will remain. Let's carefully select what works for us and enjoy the benefits of each tool we choose. What's in your toolkit today?

WHERE LOVE LIVES

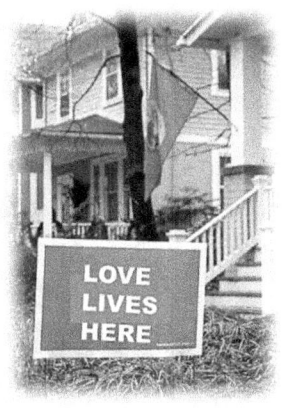

Part of our journey on this planet is discovering where love lives for us. For Kim Morton, married with two children, the discovery of where love lives pulled her out of a state of anxiety and depression that were creating panic attacks. When she decided to share how distressed she was, there was an immediate response of support from family, friends and her community. One evening a neighbor across the street texted asking her to come outside. A string of lights was attached from their side of the street to hers offering her support. Kim loved the gesture.

Other neighbors were inspired to do the same thing, and soon lights were strewn from one end of the block to the other. One neighbor made a sign from lights and coat hangers that read "LOVE LIVES HERE." Kim was so touched she was in tears. The lights kept spreading until block after block was lit up as a visible sign of everyone's connectedness and support. People from other neighborhoods came to view the lights and learn the story. The local newspaper became involved and asked Kim to share her story which she titled "Love Lives Here": the story of the lights in Rodgers Forge.[20] The lights and love helped Kim during her time of darkness and tangibly showed her where love lives. Love is in both the darkness and the light.

All of us make our way through loss and new beginnings. Love lives at the bedside of illness, it lives in compassionate medical staff, it's in the person that cleans our home, makes us a meal or provides transportation to an appointment. Love lives in the celebration of life for someone who has passed on. Love lives in every crisis. Love also lives in starting a new job, celebrating a new stage of life or getting together with friends. Love lives wherever people lift each other up and whenever we accept ourself just the way we are.

Love lives in the ordinary. It lives in backyard picnics, paying bills, folding laundry and grocery shopping. It lives in oil changes, budget adjustments, hugs and pizza nights. Love lives whether life feels heavy or light. For me loved lived in a sales person that helped me find just what I needed to wear after surgery, the nurse that held my hand when a test became painful, and the mechanic who checked out a peculiar noise in my car without charging me.

Love lives where we are most vulnerable. It lives wherever kindness is seen and compassion is shown. Love is the greatest power on earth and is needed now more than ever. No matter how chaotic the world looks, love can still live in each one of us. Finally, when we are truly listening to life, we find in our true heart of hearts our own longing to be loved, acknowledged, and understood. As Paula Hardin writes, "The wise ones all agree: Love is the most fundamental, most creative power in the world. ..... Those who have walked in love for a long time tell us this: realize that we are already within love as the fish are already in the sea. It may seem surprising, but love surrounds us and permeates us; we needn't search for it. Love is the life of our hearts and the "why" of life. When we solidly find the path of love, our lives begin to portray the highest kind of human being, one who reflects divine beauty."[21]The following poem sums this up well.

WHERE LOVE LIVES by Jenna Genevieve[22]

I imagine

That there is a place

Where love takes hold

Of even the darkest spaces.

Where peace gently roots itself

Among chaos

And confusion.

Where kindness

Softens the ground

That hasn't seen rain in months.

Where gentleness

Calms the storm

And always says "come home,"

Where life flows

Through the roughest

Of waters.

I imagine

That this place

Would be most powerful

If it found its home

In me.

We can choose to be the reservoirs of love for ourself, others, the earth with all its canyons and creatures. Love can be found in the middle of illness, heartache, loss, and confusion, as well as peacefulness, satisfying work and contentment. The choice is ours. Let's choose to be where love lives, and listen to life.

Until Next Time – Sylvia

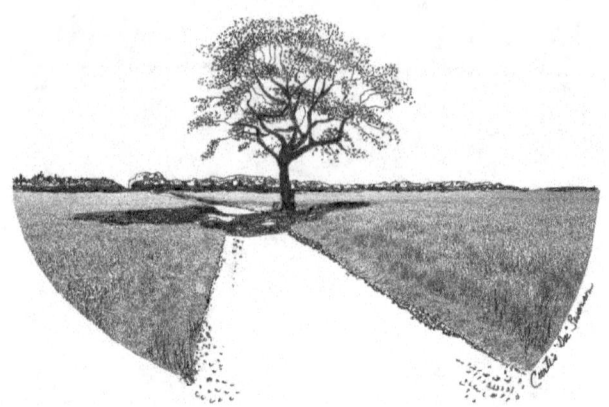

ENDNOTES

CHAPTER 1 Nature

[1] Melton,G.D., http://www.oprah.com/inspiration/glennon-doyle-melton-how-to-overcome-rock-bottom#ixzz68NPbV1OG

[2] Axner, Marya, *"Building Community Relationships: Part 1"*, Section 7. Building and Sustaining Relationships. Jodi Schultz, Moderator, Michigan State University – January 9, 2013

[3] Harbinger, A.J., www.theartofcharm.com/art-of-dating/science-eye-contact-attraction/

[4] Anderson, Sam, , Article – "The Truth About Cocoons", New York Times Magazine, May 20, 2020

[5] Williamson, Marianne, www.gooodreads.com/author/quotes/17297/Marianne_Williamson

[6] Adyashanti, , "Falling Into Grace", adyashanti.org

[7] Tolle, Eckhart, *A New Earth: Awakening to Your Life's Purpose*, PLUME, Penguin Group, New York, NY, 2006, p. 223

[8] Tolle, E, quotecatalog.com/quote/eckhart-tolle-it-is-through-t-x1mZl47

[9] Thurman, Howard, *Meditations of the Heart* (Beacon Press: 1999), 123-124.

[10] Tolle,Eckhart,www.twitter.com/EckhartTolle/status/1595601849473634304

[11] Vreeland, Susan, www.goodreads.com/quotes/6767324-no-matter

[12] Gessner, David, Quoted in "Your Brain on Nature: Finding Harmony When Human Moments Are Sparse", Article by Fran Benedict, August 20, 2020

[13] Dienstman, Allison, , "10 Unexpected Benefits of Spending Time in Nature", March 24, 2019

[14] Milton, John P., www.azquotes.com/author/10164-John_Milton

[15] Tolle, Eckhart, , *Stillness Speaks*, Namaste Publishing, Vancouver, BC, Canada, 2003, p. 82

[16] Simons, Bronwyn, , Weekly Horoscope from the Astrology Hub Podcast, Astrologer Bronwyn Simons and Amanda 'Pua' Walsh

[17] O'Neall, Margret A., ., "Facing Into the Wind" presented to the Unitarian Universalist Congregation on Sunday, April 7, 2019.

CHAPTER 2 - Inspiration

[1] Graham, Brendan, https:// en.wikipedia.org/wiki/You_Raise_Me_Up

[2] Ingersoll, Robert, https://www.goodreads.com/quotes/8119455-we-rise-by-lifting-others

[3] Meyer, Joyce, Battlefield of the Mind: Winning the Battle in Your Mind, www.goodreads.com/quotes/405354

[4] Stovall, Jim, , www.azquotes.com/quote/408953

[5] Mortman, Doris, www.goodreads.com/quotes/112887

[6] Figueroa, Tyler Butler, *America's Got Talent*,

[7] Harvey, Mandy, https://mandyharveymusic.com

[8] Kennedy, John F.,www.brainyquote.com/quotes/john_f_kennedy_103820

[9] Rinehart, Mary R., www.azquotes.com/quote/766620

[10] Reagon, Bernice Johnson, , www.goodreads.com/quotes/51340-

[11] Meshorer, Sean, https://www.seanmeshorer.com/what-is-bliss

[12] Emerson, Ralph Waldo, www.goodreads.com/quotes/1200032-the-definition-of-success--to-laugh-

[13] Girard, Joe, www.goodreads.com/quotes/26980

[14] Henson, Jim, , https://muppet.fandom.com/wiki/Jim_Henson_characters

[15] Pascal, Blaise, https://quotefancy.com/quote/776490/Blaise-Pascal

[16] White, Anna, www.goodreads.com/quotes/1046820

[17] O'Donohue, John, https://www.bing.com/videos/riverview/relatedvideo?q=John+O%27Donohue+quote%2c+"that+deep+within+each+of+us+is+an+unprotected+place+where+beauty+always+dwells"&mid=1FF49B5E2866532323A01FF49B5E2866532323A0&FORM=VIRE

[18] Adams, Thomas, www.inspiringquotes.us/author/9512-thomas-adams

[19] Myss, Caroline, *Sacred Contracts: Awakening Your Divine Potential*, Harmony, The Random House Group, New York, NY, 2003

[20] Lamott, Anne, https://goodreads.com/quotes/6476160

[21] Adams, Thomas, Lyrics to song: *Amazing Grace*

[22] Nepo, Mark, ww.internetpillar.com/mark-nepo-quotes/#:text=Keep%20the%20colors,wet.%20~%20Mark%20Nepo

[23] Rohr, Richard, *Falling Upward*, Jossey-Bass Publishing, San Francisco, CA, 2011

[24] Hawkins, David R., https://femininefierce.wordpress.com/2011/09/15

[25] Bell, Alexander G.,https://brainyquote.com/quotes/alexander_graham_bell_408695

[26] Saint-Exupery, Antoine, *The Little Prince*, Published 1943

[27] Beecher, Henry Ward, *"Life Thoughts"*, Gathered from the Extemporaneous Discourses of Henry Ward Beecher by One of His Congregation. Notes taken of Beecher's sermons by Edna Dean Proctor. Boston: Phillips, Sampson and Company, 1858

[28] Burroughs, John, .goodreads.com/author/quotes/43560.John_Burroughs

[29] Morin, Amy, *13 Things Mentally Strong People Don't Do* ,: Verywell Mind, 2014; Psychotherapist and the host of The Verywell Mind Podcast

[30] https:// www.goodreads.com/quotes/93512-you-may-encounter-many-defeats-but-you-must-not-be

31 Kassem, Suzy, www.goodreads.com/quotes/7480887

32 Bell, Rob, https://quotefancy.com/quote/1934497

33 Murat, Mehmet, https://quotefancy.com/quote/1934497

34 Breathnach, Sarah B., www.joydetectives.com/blog/tag
/Sarah+Ban+Breathnach

35 Breathnach, Sarah B., www.brainyquote.com/authors/sarah-ban-breathnach-quotes

36 Odom Jr., Leslie, www.goodreads.com/work/quotes/56789653

37 Black, Meg, https://megblack.com

38 Oxenreider, Tsh, from her blog "The Art of the Simple",
/www.theartofsimple.net

CHAPTER 3 – Insights Into Ourselves

1 Hathaway, Katherine Butler.,www.goodreads.com/author/
quotes/389496. Katharine_Butler_Hathaway

2 Breathnach, Sarah Ban, https:// www.azquotes.com/author/37895
Sarah_Ban_Breathnach

3 Perron, Mari, *A Course of Love – Book One*, Take Heart Publications,
Nevada City, CA, 2014, p.145

4 Walker, Alice, www.goodreads.com/quotes/15083-the-most-common-way-people-give-up-their-power-is

5 Eisenberg, Larry, www.heartlight.org/cgishl/quotemeal.cgi?day=20230329

6 Peace Pilgrim, www.azquotes.com/author/11673-Peace_Pilgrim

7 Leatherman, Nichole, https://chopra.com/articles/how-music-relieves-stress-and-helps-you-relax

8 Lesser, Marc, https://www.youtube.com/watch?v=aUqL2p94XMc

9 Paquette, Jonah, *Awestruck*, Shambhala Publishing, Boulder, CO, 2020, 45

10 Paquette, Jonah, Ibid, 110

11 Dalai Lama, https://www.quotesgeeks.com/dalai-lama-quotes-health/

12 Tolle, Eckhart, *A New Earth: Awakening to Your Life's Purpose*, PLUME,
Penguin Group, New York, NY, 2006, p. 102

13 Oliver, Mary, https://www.healingbrave.com/blogs/all/21-mary-oliver-quotes-about-nature

14 Kubler-Ross, Elizabeth, www.brainyquote.com/ quotes/
elisabeth_kublerross_553966

15 Tolle, Eckhart, *The Power of Now: A Guide to Spiritual Enlightenment*
,Namaste Publishing, Sheridan, WY, 1997,
https://goodreads.com/quotes/268749-any-action-is-often-better-than-no-action

16 Rumi, https://www.goodreads.com/ quotes /10201326-if-light-is-in-your-heart-you-will-find-your

[17] Brown, Brene, www.goodreads.com/quotes/433293-imperfections-are-not-inadequacies

[18] Biles, Simone, https://www. sportingnews.com/us/athletics/news/simone-biles-mental-health-athletes/2wda61k16m84zzjgam0iz7ye

[19] O'Donohue, John, www. goodreads.com/quotes/512278-when-you-become-vulnerable-any-id.....

[20] Black Elk, www. azquotes.com/quote/594929

[21] Breathnach, Sarah Ban, **Simple Abundance**, Grand Central Publishing, New York, NY, 2019, p.233

[22] Thich Nhat Hanh, www. goodreads.com/quotes/600139-you-are-what-you-want-to-become-

[23] Hanson, Rick, Paper: "Resilient: 12 Tools For Transforming Everyday Experiences Into Lasting Happiness", https://www. medium.com/the-mission/how-accepting-your-challenges-opens-the-door-to-greater

[24] Christine Northrup, **Dodging Energy Vampires**, Hay House Inc., New York, NY, 2019

[25] Thich Nhat Hanh, Ibid

[26] Welsh, Ruth Nina, https://www. www.harleytherapy.co.uk/counselling/find-your-inner-resources.htm, August 13, 2012

[27] Merton, Thomas, https:// www.goodreads.com/quotes/855888-there-is-a-pervasive-form-of-contemporary-violence-to-which

[28] O'Donohue, John, **Eternal Echoes: Celtic Reflections on Our Yearning to Belong**, Harper Perennial, New York, NY, 2000

[29] Honoré, Carl, **In Praise of Slowness: Challenging the Cult of Speed**, Harper One, New York, NY, 2005

[30] Macdonald, George, **Creation in Christ - 22nd Edition, Abridged by George MacDonald,** Edited by Rolland Hein, Regent College Publishing, Vancouver, B.C. March 15, 2004

[31] Leschak, Peter M.,https://priscillaajacks.wordpress.com/2014/02/20/all-of-us-are-watchers-of-television-of-time-clocks-of-traffic-on-the-freeway-but-few-are-observers-e

[32] Elkins, James, **The Object Stares Back** , HarperOne, New York, NY, 1997

[33] Elkins, James, Ibid

[34] Thruber, James, https://www. goodreads.com/quotes/177963-let-us-not-look-back-to-the-past-with

[35] Tolle, Eckhart, www.goodreads.com/author/quotes/4493.Eckhart_Tolle, **The Power of Now: A Guide to Spiritual Enlightenment** ,Namaste Publishing, Sheridan, WY, 1997,

[36] Tolle, Eckhart, Ibid

[37] Palmer, Parker, **Let Your Life Speak: Listening for the Voice of Vocation**, Jossey-Bass Publishing, San Francisco, CA, 1999

[38] Kehoe, John, ***Mind Power: Into the 21st Century***, Zoetic Publishing, Santa Cruz, CA, 1996

[39] Buechner, Fredrick, https://www.goodreads.com/quotes/158523-listen-to-your-life-see-it-for-the-fathom, From: ***Now and Then: A Memoir of Vocation***

[40] Radmacher, Mary Anne, www.goodreads.com/quotes/38657-courage-doesn-t-always-roar-sometimes-courage-is-the-little-voice

[41] Einstein, Albert, www.inspirationalstories.com/quotes/albert-einstein-the-intuitive-mind-is-a-sacred-gift/

CHAPTER 4 – Self Care

[1] Beattie, Melody, https:/www.melodybeattie.com/panic/ From the book: ***Codependent No More***, Spiegel-Grau, Random House, New York, NY, 2022

[2] Brown, Brene, https://brenebrown.com/podcast/brene-on-anxiety-calm-over-under-functioning/

[3] Germer, Christopher K., https:// goodreads.com/author/show/2849344.Christopher_K_Germer

[4] Martensson, Jonatan, https:// www.goodreads.com/quotes/7257602-feelings-are-much-like-waves-we-can-surf

[5] Written by Hal David, Composed by Burt Bacharach, Recorded by Jackie DeShannon in 1965

[6] Miline, A.A., ***The Winnie the Pooh Library***, A.A. Milne - Quotespedia.org; www.goodreads.com/quotes/6659295

[7] Dalai Lama, https://www.quotespedia.org/authors/d/dalai-lama/love-and-compassion-are-necessary-to-suvive

[8] Germer, Christopher K., Ibid

[9] Underwood, Jen, https:// jenunderwood.org/category/quotes/page/3/

[10] Tolle, Eckhart, https://www. goodreads.com/quotes/144636-sometimes-letting-things-go-is-an-act-of-far-greater

[11] Chernoff, Marc, https://www. goodreads.com/author/quotes/7391734.Marc_Chernoff

[12] Popov, Linda, https://www. psychologytoday.com/us/blog/the-clarity/201909/permission-feel

[13] The New York Times, A Special Section -***I Quit***, Sunday, February 2, 2020

[14] The New York Times, Ibid, Veronica Chambers, "My Job" p.4

[15] The New York Times, Ibid, Anna Dubenko, "Yale", p.5

[16] The New York Times, Ibid, Lisa Wells, "My Phone", p.8

[17] The New York Times, Ibid, Len Schreiner, "The Priesthood", p. 9

[18] The New York Times, Ibid, John Michael Hogue, "Buying Things", p.10

[19] The New York Times, Ibid, Iva Dixit, "My Elaborate Skin-Care Routine", p.13

[20] The New York Times, Ibid, Nathan Taylor Pemberton, "The Evangelical Church I Grew Up In", p. 6

[21] Tolle, Eckhart, *A New Earth: Awakening to Your Life's Purpose*, PLUME, Penguin Group, New York, NY, 2006, p. 45

[22] Boyes, Alice, "How to Recognize When You Don't Have to Do Something", https://www. psychologytoday.com/us/blog/in-practice/202204/how-recognize-when-you-dont-have-do-something

[23] Boyes, Alice, Ibid

[24] Haas, Susan B., *"Live a Life You Love: 7 Steps to a Healthier, Happier, More Passionate You*, Beaufort Books, New York, NY, 2010

[25] Backster, Cleve, www.archive.nytimes.com/www.nytimes.com/news/the-lives-they-lived/2013/12/21/cleve-backster/

[26] Emoto, Masaro, *The Hidden Messages in Water*, Beyond Words Publishing, Hillsboro, OR, p. 52

[27] Campbell, Donald, *The Mozart Effect*, William Morrow & Company, HarperCollins, New York, NY, September 18, 2001, p.167

[28] Harris, Andrew, MS, LPC – Primary Therapist, Blog #stayhomestayhopeful, April 7, 2020, Blog title: "Radical Acceptance in a Time of Uncertainty"

[29] Hall, Karyn, Ph.D., https://www.psychologytoday.com/gb/blog/pieces-mind/201207/radical-acceptance

[30] Jung, Carl, https://www. carljungdepthpsychologysite.blog/2020/01/29/popular-carl-jung-quotations-and-quotations-attributed-to-become

[31] Mahatma Gandhi, https://www. quotespedia.org/authors/m/mahatma-gandhi/happiness-is-when-what-you-think

[32] Paul, Margaret, www.innerbonding.com

[33] Suzuki, Ranata, www. awarebuzz.com/best-ranata-suzuki-quotes

[34] Griffin, Trudi, www. medium.com/koinonia/how-this-writer-confesses-with-her-mouth-through-her-pen-fb54230e2b8a

[35] Hara, Kenya, qz.com/quartzy/1140182/mujis-design-philosophy-is-emptiness-not-minimalism-says-kenya-hara

[36] Macdonald, George, *Creation in Christ - 22nd Edition, Abridged by George MacDonald,* Edited by Rolland Hein, Regent College Publishing, Vancouver, B.C. March 15, 2004

[37] Rossato-Bennett, Michael, Directed and produced the film documentary: *Alive Inside: A Story of Music and Memory*, January 18, 2014

[38] Giffords, Gabrielle & Mark Kelly, *Gabby – A Story of Courage and Hope*, Scribner, New York, NY, November 2011

[39] Albom, Mitch, *The Time Keeper*, Hyperion, New York, NY, 2012

[40] Kogan, Dr. Julia, Psychologist, Stress and Sleep Coaching www.drjuliakogan.com

41 Webb, Dr. Jonice, https://www.psychologytoday.com/us/blog/childhood-emotional-neglect/202204/how-learn-valuable-lifetime-skill-self-soothing, April 10, 2022

42 Jobs, Steve, *12 Quotes on Focusing On One Thing At A Time And Not Multi-Tasking,* EE Edit@rs ·April 12, 2016, www.examinedexistence.com/12-fantastic-quotes-one-thing-not-multi-tasking

43 Source unknown, twitter.com/Fact/status/1643249351462903810

44 Jameson, Storm, https://www.w.goodreads.com/author/quotes/44683.Storm_Jameson

45 Friedman, Meyer and Ray Roseman, *Type A Behavior and Your Heart*, Alfred A. Knopf Publishing, Penguin Random House, New York, NY , March 12, 1974

46 Kierkegaard, Soren, https:// philosophybreak.com/articles/kierkegaard-on-why-busy-people-are-ridiculous/

47 Voskamp, Ann, *One Thousand Gifts: A Dare to Live Fully Right Where You Are*, Harper Christian Resources, Nashville, TN,2012

48 Francis de Sales, https://www. goodreads.com/quotes/741506-never-be-in-a-hurry-do-everything-quietly-and-in

CHAPTER 5 – Life Skills

1 Srivastava, Garima, www.yourquote.in/garima-srivastava-w51/quotes

2 Brown, Brene, *Rising Strong*, Spiegel Grau, Random House, New York, NY, 2015, p.212

3 Wayne, John, www. jhumpoo.com/john-wayne-quotes-about-courage/

4 Schweitzer, Albert, meaningin.com/quotes/albert-schweitzer/23585-in-everyone----s-life

5 Marston, Ralph, www.overallmotivation.com/quotes/ralph-marston-quotes/

6 Williamson, Marianne, *The Gift of Change*, HarperCollins Publishing, New York, NY, 2004, p.14

7 Toffler, Alvin, *Future Shock*, Random House, New York, NY, 1970

8 Brown, Brene, Ibid. p. 35

9 Satir, Virginia, https:// www.goodreads.com/quotes/447403-life-is-not-the-way-it-s-supposed-to-be-it-s

10 Maxwell, John, https:// www.azquotes.com/author/9639-John_C_Maxwell/tag/difficulty

11 Hays, Edward M., https:// www.goodreads.com/author/quotes/9435.Edward_Hays

12 Coelho, Paulo, https:// www.goodreads.com/quotes/42488-the-simple-things-are-also-the-most-extraordinary-things-and

13 Hollis, Rachel, https:// millennial-grind.com/30-inspirational-quotes-from-girl-stop-apologizing-by-rachel-hollis/

14 Lombardo, Elizabeth, https:// www.psychologytoday.com/us/blog/better-than-perfect/201703/11-ways-to-overcome-procrastination#

15 Klein, Stephanie, https:// stephanieklein.com

16 O'Donohue, John, , *Eternal Echoes: Celtic Reflections on Our Yearning to Belong*, Harper Perennial, New York, NY, 2000

17 Armstrong, Kristen, https:// www.azquotes.com/author/16261-Kristin_Armstrong

18 Tan, Marilyn, https:// www.huffpost.com/entry/six-ways-to-manage-and-thrive-through-transition-and-change_b_5820408

19 O'Donohue, John, Ibid, p. 67

20 Wolff, Carina, https:// www.bustle.com/p/10-subtle-but-serious-signs-youre-on-the-wrong-life-path-need-to-make-a-change-59141

21 Frankl, Viktor, https:// www.goodreads.com/author/quotes/2782.Viktor_E_Frankl, From the book: *Man's Search for Meaning*, Beacon Press, Boston, MA, 2006; First printed in 1946

22 Beecher, Henry Ward, https:// www.goodreads.com/author/quotes/425221.Henry_Ward_Beecher#:

23 Soleil, Valerie, https:// www.learning-mind.com/start-over-again/

24 Ho, Leon, https:// www.lifehack.org/810843/how-to-start-over

25 Saviuc, Luminita, https:// www.purposefairy.com/74960/how-to-start-all-over/

26 Kor , Eva, https://www.huffpost.com/entry/a-holocaust-survivors-inspiring-answer-to-what-gives-you-hope-during-tough-times_b_6316622

27 Satir, Virginia, https:// www.goodreads.com/quotes/447403-life-is-not-the-way-it-s-supposed-to-be-it-s

28 Obama, Barack, https:// quotefancy.com/quote/3154/Barack-Obama-The-best-way-to-not-feel-hopeless-is-to-get-up-and-do-something-Don-t-wait#:

29 Goodier, Steve, https:// www.goodreads.com/quotes/691477-who-do-you-spend-time-with-criticizers-or-encouragers-surround

30 Dickenson, Emily, https://www.poetryfoundation.org/poems/42889/hope-is-the-thing-with-feathers-314

31 Katie, Byron, *A Mind at Home With Itself*, HarperOne, New York, NY, 2018

32 Dalai Lama, https://www.quotespedia.org/authors/d/dalai-lama/when-you-talk-you-are-only-repeating-what-you-already-know-but-if-you-listen-you-may-learn-something

33 Saviuc, Luminita, From the book: *15 Things You Should Give Up to Be Happy: An Inspiring Guide to Discovering Effortless Joy*, https:// www.goodreads.com/author/quotes/8120065.Luminita_D_Saviuc

[34] Lincoln, Abraham, https://www.azquotes.com/author/8880-Abraham_Lincoln

[35] Gates, Bill, https:// quoteinvestigator.com/2014/02/26/lazy-job/

[36] Franklin, Benjamin, https:// www.fi.edu/en/benjamin-franklin/famous-quotes

[37] Bailey, Chris, *Hyperfocus*, Penquin Books, New York, NY, 2019

[38] Foster, Jeffrey, www.youtube.com/watch?v=FZLhJGmpBLY

[39] Dyer, Wayne, https:// www.goodreads.com/quotes/207773-be-miserable-or-motivate-yourself-whatever-has-to-be-done

[40] *Ride Like A Girl* – Movie- Starring: Teresa Palmer , Sam Neill, Sullivan Stapleton , et al, Directed by: Rachel Griffiths

[41] Dhali Lama, https:// www.goodreads.com/quotes/24245-if-there-is-no-solution-to-the-problem-then-don-t

[42] Campbell, Joseph, https:// www.lifehack.org/articles/lifestyle/find-place-inside-where-theres-joy.html

[43] Lincoln, Abraham, https:/ /statushappy.com/quotes/836/the-best-thing-about-the-future-is-that-it-only-comes-one-day-at-a-time.

[44] Arruda, William, https://www.forbes.com/sites/williamarruda/2020/03/15/9-ways-to-stay-positive-during-the-coronavirus-pandemic/?sh=52d68baa5a8e

CHAPTER 6 – Nurturing Relationships

[1] Chef Padma Lakshmi, *Top Chef - The Cookbook*, Revised Edition, Chronicle Books, 2009

[2] www. ntsb.gov/investigations/AccidentReports/Reports/AAR8903.pdf

[3] Penn, Delores, Contributing quote, Board member of Friends After Diagnosis Cancer Support Group, Vero Beach, FL, June 12, 2020

[4] Knost, L. R., www. littleheartsbooks.com/about-the-authorillustrator/

[5] Cummings, E.E., www.graciousquotes.com/e-e-cummings/

[6] Brown, Brene, www.azquotes.com/author/19318-Brene_Brown/tag/authenticity

[7] Carter, Christine, www.greatergood.berkeley.edu/article/item/five_ways_to_be_fully_authentic

[8] Brown, Brene, *Braving the Wilderness* , Random House, New York, NY, 2017, p.63

[9] Chodron, Pema, https://www.goodreads.com/quotes/179969

[10] Nepo, Mark, *Seven Thousand Ways to Listen*, ATRIA Paperback, Simon & Schuster, New York, NY, 2013, page 84

[11] Popov, Linda, *A Pace of Grace*, Penguin Group (USA)Inc., New York, NY, 2004, page 245

[12] Rilke, Rainer Maria, www.inspirationalstories.com/quotes/rainer-maria-rilke

[13] Dyer, Wayne, www.azquotes.com/quote/589437

[14] Covey, Steven, www.quotemaster.org/qce5004d8aa3470c0592799dc8522f6d6

[15] Benedict, Fran, Vitamin "F": Forgiveness – and the Power of Letting Go, chopra.com/articles/vitamin-f-forgiveness-and-the-power-of-letting-go, July 1, 2020

[16] Winfrey, Oprah, , www.goodreads.com/quotes/376558

[17] Holub, Ann, *Forgive and Be Free*, Llewellyn Publications, Woodbury, MN, 2014

[18] Muller, Robert, ww.Goodreads.com/author/quotes/41021.Robert_Muller

[19] Ram Dass, www. ramdass.org/ram-dass-quotes/

[20] Stotts Stuart, htpps://stuartstotts.com/songlyrics/

[21] Northrup, Christine, *Dodging Energy Vampires*, Hay House Inc., Vista, CA, 2019

[22] Eadie, Betty, www.inspiringquotes.us/author/9094-betty-eadie

[23] Hurst, Katherine, , article titled, "The Power Of Words: How A Single Word Can Impact Your Life, https://www. thelawofattraction.com/the-power-of-words/

CHAPTER 7 – Holidays

[1] Jung, Carl G., https:// www.goodreads.com/quotes/1204404-one-does-not-become-enlightened-by-imagining-figures-of-light

[2] Beck, Martha, *Finding Your Own North Star: Claiming the Life You Were Meant to Live*, Harmony Publishing, Penquin Random House, New York, NY, 2002 p. 46

[3] Beck, Martha, Ibid, p. 145

[4] Whyte, David, https:// thevalueofsparrows.wordpress.com/2018/10/29/words-genius-by-david-whyte/

[5] Lombardo, Elizabeth, *A Happy You: Your Ultimate Prescription for Happiness*, Morgan James Publishing, New York, NY, 2009

[6] Williams, Don, https:// genius.com/Don-williams-take-it-easy-on-yourself-lyrics

[7] Kerr, Jolie, New York Times Article, *"How to Survive the Holidays"*, November 19, 2019

[8] Rogers, Fred, https:// www.azquotes.com/author/12542-Fred_Rogers

CHAPTER 8 – Dealing With Illness

[1] Kern, Ivanna, https:// w.mdanderson.org/cancerwise/appendix-cancer-surv.h00-159064767.html

[2] Leaper, Caroline, *32963 Newspaper*, Vero Beach 32963 Media, Vero Beach, FL, February 13, 2020

[3]Standish, Jules, *The Essential Guide to Mindful Dressing: Choose Your Colours – Control Your Life*, O-Books, John Hunt Publishing, Blue Ridge Summit, PA, 2016, p. 45, https:// www.scribd.com/book/388555505/The-Essential-Guide-to-Mindful-Dressing-Choose-your-colours-Control-your-life#:

[4] Covey, Stephen, *"Seven Habits of Highly Effective People"*, Simon & Schuster, New York, NY, 2020, https:// www.forbes.com/sites/kevinkruse/2012/07/16/the-7-habits/?sh=1dea2aa739c6

[5] Field, Rick, Rick Field, son of actor Sally Field, is a physicist at the University of Florida and part of the CMS collaboration at the Large Hadron Collider. He is known for his contributions to the phenomenology of particle production in high-energy particle accelerators.

[6] Irion, Mary Jean, https:// www.goodreads.com/quotes/101242-normal-day-let-me-be-aware-of-the-treasure-you

[7] Kimbrough, Emily, https://www.goodreads.com/author/quotes/147203.Emily_Kimbrough#

[8] Steindl-Rast, David, https://quotefancy.com/quote/1511015/David-Steindl-Rast-As-I-express-my-gratitude-I-become-more-deeply-aware-of-it-And-the

[9] Beattie, Melody, https:// www.goodreads.com/quotes/67563-gratitude-unlocks-the-fullness-of-life-it-turns-what-we

[10] Palmer, Parker, https:// quotefancy.com/quote/1510330/Parker-J-Palmer-I-will-always-have-fears-but-I-need-not-be-my-fears-for-I-have-other

[11] Nepo, Mark, https:// www.goodreads.com/work/quotes/10685-the-book-of-awakening-having-the-life-you-want-by-being-present-to-the

[12] Beattie, Melody, https:// www.goodreads.com/author/quotes/4482.Melody_Beattie

[13] Nepo, Mark, https:// www.goodreads.com/author/quotes/ 5136 .Mark_Nepo

[14] Wu, Jade, https:// www.quickanddirtytips.com/articles/7-simple-tips-to-help-you-stop-feeling-inadequate/#:~:text=7%20Simple%20Tips%20to

[15] Elliot, T.S., https:// ww.treasurequotes.com/quotes/the-journey-not-the-arrival-matters-2#:~

[16] Williams, Serena, https:// www.goodreads.com/author/quotes/157634 .Serena_Williams#:~:

17 Gucciardi, Anthony, https:// anthonygucciardi.com/mindset/17-powerful-quotes-to-help-you-get-through-hard-times/

18 DeGeneres, Ellen, https:// www.goodreads.com/quotes/138766-procrastination-is-not-the-problem-it-is-the-solution-it#:~:

19 Newhouse, Leo, https:// www.health.harvard.edu/blog/is-crying-good-for-you-2021030122020#:

20 Morton, Kim, https:// www.baltimoresun.com/opinion/op-ed/bs-ed-op-1225-rodgers-forge-lights-20201224-br6hum6dxngxdgpwcbqgn2ce6a-story.html

21 Hardin, Paula Payne, *Love After Love – Stages of Loving*, New World Library, Novato, CA, 1996, p.28

22 Genevieve, Jenna, *"Where Love Lives"*, https://jennagenevieve.blog, February 27, 2020

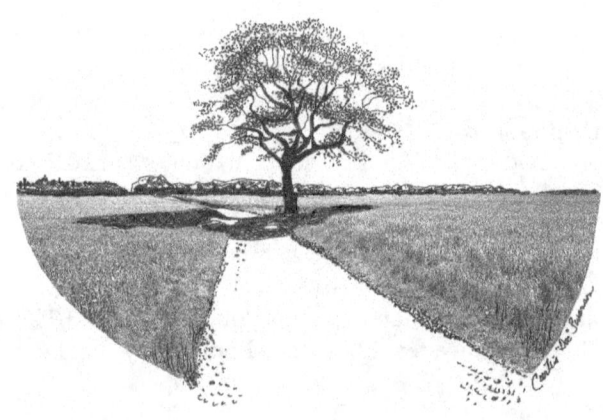

Acknowledgements

Every writer knows a book involves more than just the author. My gratitude extends first to Lynn Reading and Larry Macke who were the voice of support and encouragement to continue writing by offering needed advice and guidance. They were the founders of the Friends After Diagnosis* cancer support group that was helpful to me during my cancer experience. I learned so much from you both. Thank you for offering me the opportunity to write on your website.

Next, I want to thank my sister, Paula Hardin, whose expertise as a published author of two books herself enabled her to give me a significant editorial contribution. She also listened as I shared ideas and gave me tactful honest feedback. Our children and grandchildren have been totally supportive with plenty of hugs and positive energy.

My deepest thanks belong to my husband Curt who gave me uninterrupted writing time, made nourishing meals, read everything I wrote and did the artwork and illustrations throughout the book. He also spent long hours on computer layout and organization of the text. His editing suggestions improved my writing and his constant support was an inspiration. You are the best!

Thank you to you my readers for taking time to peruse this book. May you know how precious you really are.

* https://www.facebook.com/friendsafterdiagnosis/
*https://www.friendsafterdiagnosis.com

About the Author

Sylvia was born in Illinois and spent summers in Wisconsin where she met her husband. They have two grown children, five grandchildren and one great grandchild. Sylvia uses her life experience of working through her own tough life challenges to reach out to others who are struggling. She did this through teaching high school (she was teacher of the year twice), working with people in crisis, being a Guardian Ad Litem for five years, helping with equestrian therapy classes, and walking beside women going through cancer.

Sylvia and her husband had the opportunity to live in England for three years while her husband taught at a downtown London university. They took that opportunity to travel to many different countries experiencing different cultures. That experience confirmed for Sylvia the importance of welcoming change, valuing diversity, and discovering the common denominators in our humanity.

Her own cancer experience was in 2014 and this is when she learned that cancer recovery isn't just about feeling broken, but about being broken open to inner healing beyond cancer. Grateful for the benefit of a cancer support group, she now writes bimonthly blog articles for their website to offer support and encouragement. This book is a collection of those articles because they not only apply to people with cancer but anyone interested in making the most of life's challenges by listening to life.

For Sylvia writing from the heart is the key to connecting to the world around us, so this is from her heart to yours. May you feel the love and support within these pages.

www.ingramcontent.com/pod-product-compliance
Lightning Source LLC
Chambersburg PA
CBHW060909120626
46553CB00001B/267